Mini-Med: The Role of Regional Campuses in U.S. Medical Education

William T. Mallon
Mandy Liu
Robert F. Jones
Michael Whitcomb

Published by the
Association of American Medical Colleges

Copyright © 2003 by the Association of American Medical Colleges.

All rights reserved. No part of this publication may be reproduced, stored in a retrieval system, or transmitted, in any form or by any means, electronic, mechanical, photocopying, recording, or otherwise, without the prior written permission of the Association of American Medical Colleges.

Library of Congress Cataloging-in-Publication Data

Mini-Med: The Role of Regional Campuses in U.S. Medical Education/ William T. Mallon..[et al.].

    p. cm.
Includes bibliographical references and index
ISBN 1-57754-026-3
1. Medical colleges–Decentralization–United States   I. Mallon, William T. (Williams Thomas), 1969-
R745.M617 2003
610'. 71'173–dc21   2003005156

Available from:
Association of American Medical Colleges
Section for Publication Orders
2450 N Street NW, Washington DC 22037-1134
Phone: (202) 828-0416   Fax: (202) 828-1123
www.aamc.org/publications

Member price: $20 (Item code: MM)
Non-member price: $27 (Item code: MMN)

Contents

Acknowledgements.................................. ii

1. Introduction 1

2. History and Context............................... 5

3. Methods 17

4. An Overview of the Clinical Branch Campuses at
   U.S. Medical Schools 23

5. Why a Regional Clinical Campus? 33

6. Medical Student Education at the Regional Campus 37

7. The Organizational Relationships Between Main Campus
   and Branch Campus............................... 51

8. Conclusions....................................... 63

Appendices 65

References 83

Index... 87

Acknowledgements

We would like to acknowledge the Josiah Macy, Jr. Foundation whose generous support made this study possible. We also acknowledge the many medical school deans, associate deans for medical education, regional campus deans, administrators, faculty members, and students who participated in this study by completing surveys, participating in interviews and focus groups, and compiling written documentation. We are especially grateful to the ten regional clinical campuses that hosted us for site visits:

Mercer University School of Medicine, Savannah Campus

SUNY Upstate Medical University, Binghamton campus

Tufts University School of Medicine, Baystate Medical Center campus

UMDNJ Robert Wood Johnson Medical School, Camden campus

University of Alabama School of Medicine, Huntsville campus

University of Arizona College of Medicine, Phoenix campus

UCSF School of Medicine, Fresno campus

University of Florida College of Medicine, Jacksonville campus

University of Oklahoma College of Medicine, Tulsa campus

West Virginia University School of Medicine, Charleston campus

1. INTRODUCTION

What is a medical school? Traditionally, two notions come to mind. First, a medical school is a *concept*: an organized and unified curriculum of medical education that prepares students to be physicians. Second, a medical school is a physical *place*, a campus of classrooms and laboratories and hospitals. It is a space of defined boundaries, even if, at times, the lines between the school and the hospital or clinic might be blurred.

With more and more educational opportunities found in ambulatory settings and distributed hospitals, the modern concept of the medical school defies a campus boundary. The medical school is the main campus, to be sure, but it is also its outpatient settings in the suburbs, its inner-city clinics, and its affiliated hospitals down the road and across town. So, the medical school is, now, a broad geographic location as much as a specific university campus.

But for 20 percent of the medical schools in the United States, the idea of the medical school even transcends this confined geographic framework. At these institutions, the medical school is not only in Tucson or San Francisco or Oklahoma City or Birmingham but also in Phoenix and Fresno and Tulsa and Tuscaloosa. For 25 of our nation's medical schools, soon to be 27, the medical school is at least two campuses, not one: it is the main campus plus one or more regional clinical campuses. Significant portions of third-year (and sometimes fourth-year) medical students receive their clinical training at these branch sites. These campuses have a chief administrative officer (the "regional dean") and administrative staff; full-time, part-time, and volunteer faculty members; student support and services; and, sometimes, on-campus housing. The regional deans can be responsible not only for the clinical education program but also for facilities and physical plant, clinical services, research, contracting, and other administrative duties. These campuses are, in effect, "mini" medical schools, lacking only basic science instruction.

Yet little is known about these places. Why do they exist? How do they work? What experiences do students have there? What challenges do campus administrators face?

These questions are more than academic and the answers should interest more than just those leaders who manage schools with clinical campuses. The academic medicine community should focus on these campuses for two important and timely reasons. First, the clinical campus model is part of a larger "distributed" method of clinical education. It demands an understanding of the relationships of the site to the "parent" school. All medical schools that use multiple hospitals and ambulatory settings for clinical education will be interested in the challenges of managing and leading in the distributed model.

Second, as society debates the nation's physician supply and as medical schools consider increasing class size, clinical campuses deserve a detailed examination. What if policy makers determine that an increase in the number of physicians is desirable? Given the cost of new facilities and other constraints, an unlikely response would be to create a large contingent of new medical schools, as was the case in the 1960s. Rather, the increased use of existing clinical campus sites and the addition of new clinical campuses would seem to be a cost-effective and likely model for expansion.

Genesis of this Study

This study on regional clinical campuses has several geneses. It is a direct outgrowth of the AAMC Project on the Clinical Education of Medical Students. Conducted in 2000-01 with support from the Josiah Macy, Jr. Foundation, the AAMC Project conducted a comprehensive review of the clinical education of medical students in order to affect changes in the design and conduct of the clinical curriculum. One of the investigators' unanticipated findings was that at schools with clinical campuses, the fourth-year students who had attended those regional sites consistently praised the experience. Because a more thorough study of regional campuses was not part of the Project's design, its principal investigator recommended a follow-up study.

At the same time, the chief administrative officers at the clinical campuses—the "regional deans"—petitioned the governance of the AAMC to form a professional development group within the Association's framework. However, little was known about the number of clinical campuses and the scope of responsibilities of these regional deans.

Because of these two developments, the AAMC's Division of Medical Education and the Division of Medical School Services and Studies collaborated on the study described herein.

What is a Regional Clinical Campus?

The goals of this project were to investigate and analyze the structure, organization, operations, and management of clinical campuses. But what is a clinical campus?

These sites are called by many names: regional, branch, satellite, geographically separate. We will use these terms interchangeably in this report. However, we only focus on clinical campuses where third- and fourth-year medical students are educated. A number of medical schools also have regional basic science campuses (see appendix 1); these sites are *not* included in this study.

Several existing definitions of regional campuses informed our study. The Liaison Committee on Medical Education defines a "geographically separated campus" as "a branch campus that is geographically remote but under the central administrative or program governance of the medical school." A recent unpublished report by an AAMC scholar-in-residence suggested a regional campus has the following characteristics:

1. The site is located more than 50 miles away from the main academic health center or school of medicine

2. The site is designed so that students receive a significant component of their education at the site, whether in the basic sciences or clinical years. This must be distinguished from sites at which students rotate only a few weeks for a single clerkship experience (for example, family medicine);

3. The site has a formal administrative and educational relationship with the school of medicine. (Swick, 2000)

An unpublished study by a consultant group (Watt et al., 1993) identified regional campuses "as ones in which a medical school offers significant concentrations of basic science, clinical clerkship, and/or residency training in communities 'at a distance' from the main medical school campuses" (p. iii). Their definition was bounded by a number of exclusions:

> Excluded from this definition are: (1) the more common situation in which a medical school provides training at multiple hospitals in the same metropolitan area as its main campus; (2) situations where multiple medical schools are governed and report through a single state university administrative structure; and (3) medical schools that have developed even more decentralized programmatic initiatives, such as rural primary care preceptorships, rather than clusters of programs geographically separated from its main site. (Watt et al., 1993, p. iii)

Finally, in its Part II questionnaire, the LCME defines a "major" hospital affiliate as:

> An institution [that] is an important part of the teaching program of the medical school and is a major site of the clinical clerkship program. In general, major teaching institutions provide clerkship experience in two or more of the major services, i.e., internal medicine, surgery, pediatrics, obstetrics/gynecology. An institution responsible for most of the teaching in a single specialty, such as psychiatry or pediatrics, may also be considered a major affiliate. A major teaching affiliate is regularly used as a site of inpatient teaching for clinical clerkships. Students are under the direct supervision of medical school faculty members. A major teaching affiliate may or may not be used for residency training by the medical school.

For purposes of this study, we wanted to investigate sites that were more complex than "major" hospital affiliates. There are hundreds of major hospital affiliates but most offer limited duration experiences, typically in a nearby location to the medical school, without a tie to the dean's office. We wanted to insure that a medical school "culture" existed at the regional site. On the other hand, we did not want to arbitrarily set a limit on geographic distance. Therefore, we defined a clinical campus as meeting three criteria:

1. The campus is geographically separate and does not serve as the medical school's primary clinical site for medical student education.
2. The campus has an administrative tie to the office of the dean (not only with departmental ties).
3. The campus offers four of the required third-year clerkships.

Using this definition, we identified 41 regional campuses at 25 medical schools. (More information can be found in the Methods section, page 17.) Additionally, three schools were in the process of opening new regional campuses at the time of our study: University of Texas, San Antonio Medical School opened a branch in Harlingen in July 2002; Virginia Commonwealth University School of Medicine is planning a clinical campus in Fairfax, to open in 2005; and West Virginia University School of Medicine will open a campus in Martinsburg in approximately 2007.

2. HISTORY AND CONTEXT

An essential part of our study was to understand the historical context for the growth of regional campuses at U.S. medical schools as well as the previous research on regional campuses, community-based medical education, and multi-campus universities. First, this section undertakes a historical review of why regional campuses developed in the latter part of the twentieth century. Second, we review the relevant literature to set our study in the proper research context.

HISTORICAL INFLUENCES ON THE DEVELOPMENT OF REGIONAL CAMPUSES

The history of medical education in the second half of the twentieth century is well documented (e.g., Ludmerer, 1999). None of these historical reviews, however, gives much scholarly attention to the growth of regional campuses. Perhaps such oversight is unsurprising; these campuses seem to have developed under the radar and other events have had more immediate or significant impact on the current state of medical education.

A review of the historical antecedents and context of clinical campus, however, is important. There are at least seven separate trends or events that influenced the growth and understanding of clinical campuses. We will examine each.

The Physician Shortage of the 1960s

Official endorsements from various groups to increase the physician supply in the United States began in the 1950s. The AAMC issued a statement at its 1956 annual meeting that the country "should increase its output of physicians by increasing the number of its medical schools" (AAMC, 1958, p. 56). In 1959, a consultant group to the Surgeon General released *Physicians for a Growing America* (also called the Bane Report), which argued that the nation was heading for a severe physician shortage by 1975. It decried the lack of opportunity in many states for qualified students to attend medical school. To solve this problem, the group argued that the country should expand its current medical schools and create new ones to increase physician production.

Physicians for a Growing America was the most influential report on medical education since Flexner (Ludmerer, 1999). It provided the momentum to pass the Health Professions Education Assistant Act of 1963 (P.L. 88-129). The law authorized matching grants to assist in building new teaching facilities or rehabilitate existing facilities provided that medical schools raise their class size by five percent or by five students. The act also created a student loan fund for up to $2,000 per academic year. Further federal legislation in 1965, 1968, and in the 1970s provided additional financial incentives for medical schools to increase class size.

And they did. Nationwide, first-year enrollment increased 74 percent between 1963 and 1975, from 8,772 to 15,295. The number of fully accredited MD programs increased from 83 to 109 in the same period (Robinson, 2002).

Another influential report was released in 1970. The Carnegie Commission on Higher Education addressed the physician shortage in *Higher Education and the Nation's Health.* It asserted, "the United States today faces only one serious manpower shortage, and that is in health care personnel" (p. 2). It recommended increasing the number of first-year medical students by 50 percent—to 16,400—by 1978. It proposed a "health care delivery" model of health training that "needs to be located where people live" (p. 6), and argued for the creation of nine new university health science centers.

In both the Bane Report and the Carnegie Report, some recommendations were heeded and met, and other goals were not. The targets for first-year matriculants to medical schools in both reports were realized. The Bane Report set a goal of 15,000 first-year students by 1975. That year, 15,295 enrolled. The Carnegie Report's call for 16,400 by 1978 was surpassed slightly with an actual enrollment in that year of 16,501.

Medical schools devised alternative solutions to other recommendations. Only one of the nine cities identified in the Carnegie Report for a new health science center and medical school actually developed one (Eastern Virginia Medical School in Norfolk.) Another became an accredited two-year school (Duluth, Minnesota). No program developed in a third city (Wilmington, Delaware). But, very interestingly, the remaining six cities identified in the Carnegie Report—Phoenix, Arizona; Springfield, Massachusetts; Jacksonville, Florida; Tulsa, Oklahoma; Fresno, California; and Wichita, Kansas—eventually become home to a regional clinical campus rather than a new university health science center.

Policy makers acted quickly and forcefully to the various reports on physician manpower. The actual outcomes, however, did not always match the idealized solutions. In some states, rather than build a new medical school, officials opened branch campuses to increase clinical training opportunities for medical students, allowing them to increase class size. That six of the nine cities slated for new medical schools in the 1970 Carnegie Report developed, instead, regional branch campuses underscores the difficulties in starting new medical schools: high start-up costs; local and state politics; turf battles among universities; and the reluctance of existing medical schools for new competition.

As part of the concern over the number of physicians in the country, policy makers and the public issued specific alarms about the distribution of general and specialty physicians. As part of the reauthorization of the Health Professions Education Assistance Act in 1976, Congress attended to this concern as well. The 1976 bill increased the number of residency positions in primary care areas of family practice, internal medicine, and pediatrics. Medical schools, in turn, had increased financial incentive to develop new programs or affiliate with existing residency programs in primary care.

Six of the ten regional campuses that we visited for this study were started in the 1970s. Of this group, each had its genesis, in part, because of the national discussion of physician shortages. As already mentioned, Fresno, Tulsa, and Jacksonville were cited in the 1970 Carnegie Report. Some campuses explicitly tied their mission to the physician shortage and, more explicitly, to the need for primary care physicians. For example, a 1973 study for the New York Regents identified Binghamton and environs as a physician shortage area. Therefore, SUNY Upstate Medical University's proposal to develop a clinical campus in Binghamton asserted it would provide "the educational loci which could assist in the recruitment and retention of primary care physicians in the area, especially rural counties" and would expose "medical students to the satisfaction and rewards of primary care practices in rural segments of the area" (qtd. in SUNY, 1990).

The "Right" to Health Care

Regional campuses have their geneses in several other movements of the post-World War II era. Another was the belief that access to health care was a universal right, a concept institutionalized when Congress enacted the Medicare program in 1965 (Lewis & Sheps, 1983). By 1970, the

Carnegie Commission would write, "increasingly, health care is coming to be regarded not only as a necessity but also as a right to which all persons are entitled" (p. 15). In this milieu, academic medical centers were viewed as the best sources of medical care. Therefore, "the philosophy underlying postwar federal health policy was that each region of the country should be served by one or more major teaching hospitals, which would provide consultations to smaller hospitals in the region and specialized hospital care to any patient in the region who needed it" (Ludmerer, 1999, p. 164).

The Carnegie Report reflected this view. It argued that university health science centers have an important role in each state or region to help communities "develop model health care systems" (p. 46) and cooperate "with other community agencies in improving the organization of health care delivery" (p. 47). The Commission proposed 126 area health education centers (AHECs) to serve localities without a medical school. These centers would be administered by the university health science center, train medical students and residents on a rotational basis, run continuing education programs for local physicians, and contribute to the improvement of heath care in the region.

To meet the need of improved access to high-quality care, the federal government provided funding for new programs. As recommended by the Carnegie Commission, the national AHEC program was established in 1972 to provide primary care services in medically underserved areas. AHECs received legal status in 1976 legislation; medical schools that received AHEC funding were required to educate at least 10 percent of their students at remote sites. Also in the 1970s, the Veteran's Administration developed affiliations with several medical schools and, through the Veteran's Administration Medical School Assistance Act of 1972, provided funds for construction of medical education facilities. In addition to the creation of five new medical schools, the 1972 VA law led to the creation of one new clinical campus, located in Fresno.

Many of the regional campuses in our study were created to respond to the health care needs of the surrounding area. When the Huntsville campus of the University of Alabama School of Medicine was authorized by the legislature in 1971, it was developed with the belief "that community-based branch campuses… produce a larger proportion of primary care physicians. The intent of the trustees was to ensure that a greater number of future UASOM graduates would practice in the primary care specialties in rural areas of the state" (Berg, 2002, p. 3). A consultant's report from 1973 on the

UCSF Fresno campus cited a similar goal: "An immediate impact of the program will be to improve the overall level of health care services available to the people residing in the Central San Joaquin Valley."

The Move of Medical Practice to Ambulatory Settings

A third historical influence on the development of clinical campuses was the changing delivery of medical care. As Ludmerer (1999) summarizes, inpatient facilities had been a source of excellent learning opportunities for the first half of the 20th century. But as tertiary teaching hospitals focused more on complex cases, community hospitals were needed for "bread and butter" teaching. Technological advances and pharmaceutical therapies pushed routine surgical and psychiatry cases into outpatient settings. Advances in health care made hospital stays shorter and less necessary. These changes in health care led one observer to conclude "during the early 1980s, no medical school in the United States or Canada had been able to implement the full spectrum of its educational programs for the physician in a single teaching hospital" (Schofield, 1984, p. 218).

These changes, coupled with increased class size, affected the ability of medical schools to provide adequate clinical experiences to their students. In turn, many developed affiliations with other hospitals.

> The increased number of students assigned as clinical clerks in the teaching hospitals, together with an expanded corps of hospital residents and clinical fellows, congested these institutions and thus diluted each student's "hands on" experience with patients. To cope with the crowded conditions and the need to provide students with a solid clinical education, most schools were forced to extend their teaching activities into more and more affiliated, community, and veterans hospitals.... In some instances, however, branch campuses were developed—sometimes at a considerable distance from the site of the medical school and the faculty based there. (Schofield, 1984, p. 46)

Many of the ten regional sites visited in our study were founded because of the need for additional clinical capacity. Tufts' campus at Baystate Medical Center in Springfield, Arizona's Phoenix campus, Mercer's Savannah campus, UMDNJ's Camden campus, and Florida's Jacksonville campus, for example, all started because, among other reasons, the need for expanded clinical teaching opportunities.

The Expansion of Graduate Medical Education

A fourth influence on the creation of clinical campuses, related to the changes in medical practice, was the expansion of graduate medical education opportunities in postwar America. As the number of residents and fellows expanded over the years, so did the need for more patients for teaching purposes. Therefore, "many schools expanded their clinical network beyond their original teaching hospital to establish affiliations with veterans hospitals, municipal hospitals, specialty hospitals, and selected community hospitals…" (Ludmerer, 1999, p. 184). The number of freestanding residency programs, unaffiliated with medical schools, greatly expanded after World War II. But, as Ludmerer notes, these programs faced stiff competition. "Hospitals without a medical school affiliation often struggled to fill their allocated positions, and some could not fill even half their quota" (p. 184). The medical education program at several of the hospitals now affiliated with clinical campuses in our study began as freestanding residency programs. The first examples of medical education programs in many cities were at the graduate level. Over the years, however, these freestanding programs sought to become affiliated with the medical school because of the prestige and name recognition of a residency allied with a university medical center.

Other Contributing Influences

There were a number of other changes in the financing and organization of higher education and research in the 1960s and 1970 that affected how the emergence of regional medical education was perceived. First, the growing belief in America that access to higher education was a basic right helped create conditions for medical schools to enlarge class size. Second, the development of branch campuses and multicampus networks in universities made the idea of regional clinical campuses in medical schools seem less foreign and strange. Third, the growth of the biomedical research enterprise in the nation's medical schools created a research "culture" that equated basic research with high quality. In turn, less research-intense sites, such as community-based schools and clinical campuses, were perceived as lower quality. Each of these contributing influences will be examined in greater detail.

The "Right" to Access in Postsecondary Education

As Americans developed the belief that they have a right to high-quality healthcare, they also adopted the view that anyone should have access to a college education. Federal legislation in 1963 under the Johnson administration and continuing into the 1970s focused on equal opportunity and greatly expanded student aid programs. The 1970 Carnegie Commission report noted a similar concern for medical education when it asserted, "there is a particularly critical need for grants for student from low-income families who wish to undertake [medical] education" (p. 63).

Some champions of regional clinical education programs envisioned these sites would also enlarge access. For example, in creating the clinical medical education program in Fresno, the California State Legislature expressed its concern that "California citizens, desiring to become physicians, do not have an adequate opportunity to attend medical schools in California."

The Development of Distributed Education

Statewide systems of higher education and multi-campus universities began to form in the 1950s and 1960s with the large increases in college enrollments. The multicampus university, defined by the "coexistence of geographically distinct communities" (Lee & Bowen, 1971, p. 2), challenged the notion of the prevalent higher education model of a closed system, in which a university was defined by the discrete geographical setting of the campus. As university systems like those in California, Illinois, Maryland, Texas, and Wisconsin emerged, higher education leaders devised organizational structures to accommodate distributed teaching, governance, and administration. While the development of medical school clinical campuses is not directed linked to the creation of these multicampus systems, they are important historical antecedents to the regional campus.

The Growth in Biomedical Research

Simultaneous to the growth of the clinical enterprise and the physician shortage in the 30 years after World War II was the explosion in biomedical research. This trend is important in understanding the creation of clinical campuses for two reasons. First, it is another example of the federal government's role in the expansion of the medical school enterprise in the 1960s and 1970s. Second, because of that support, a distinctive culture of research formed at academic medical centers, which in turn has had an effect on how non-research oriented clinical campuses were perceived.

The federal government's support of biomedical research grew exponentially after World War II. The National Institutes of Health expenditure for medical research grew from $8.3 million in 1947 to $800 million in 1966 (Shannon, 1967). The launch of Sputnik in 1957 transformed university-based research (Geiger, 1993). The Seaborg Report ("Scientific Progress, the Universities, and the Federal Government"), released in 1960, crystallized the view that the federal government ought to be universities' primary source of research funding (Geiger, 1993). Medical schools benefited greatly compared to their university brethren. "By 1972, medical schools accounted for 10 percent of the total expenditures of higher education and employed about 10 percent of all personnel, even though they enrolled only about 0.5 percent of students" (Ludmerer, 1999, p. 142). The rise of NIH during this period "fixed medical schools as the most research-intensive academic component of universities" (Geiger, 1993, p. 185).

The growth in the research enterprise contributed to a culture in which research has preeminence over teaching. Burton Clark (1987) found that "teaching institutions remain all-teaching at the price of remaining in the middle or lower reaches of the [academic] hierarchy…the mark of first-class practice is the provision of considerable time for research" (pp. 99-100). Even today, popular media outlets rank the "best" medical schools and universities based on research expenditures (e.g. U.S. News and World Report), not necessarily the best teaching and learning environments. The new medical schools created in the 1960s reported difficulty being accepted by their traditional counterparts, in part, because of their preoccupation with educational issues and modest funding of research (Hunt, 1979). Many of the regional clinical campuses, which focus almost entirely on clinical teaching with little or no research enterprise, faced similar challenges.

Summary of Historical Influences

Amid a growth in population, changes in societal expectations, and advances in the practice and delivery of healthcare, the nation's academic medicine community in the 1960s and 1970s faced a number of pressures. With the advent of large-scale government-sponsored health insurance, Americans viewed access to high-quality care as their right. Policy makers and analysts warned of impending physician shortages. Students demanded equal access to all levels of higher education. More and more of medicine moved from the ward to the ambulatory setting. These influences created an environment in which medical education leaders needed to create more access to learners and more space for patients. As a result, large cadres of new medical schools were founded in the sixties and seventies. But also, while smaller in scale, a considerable number of regional campuses began in the same period for similar reasons (see figure 1).

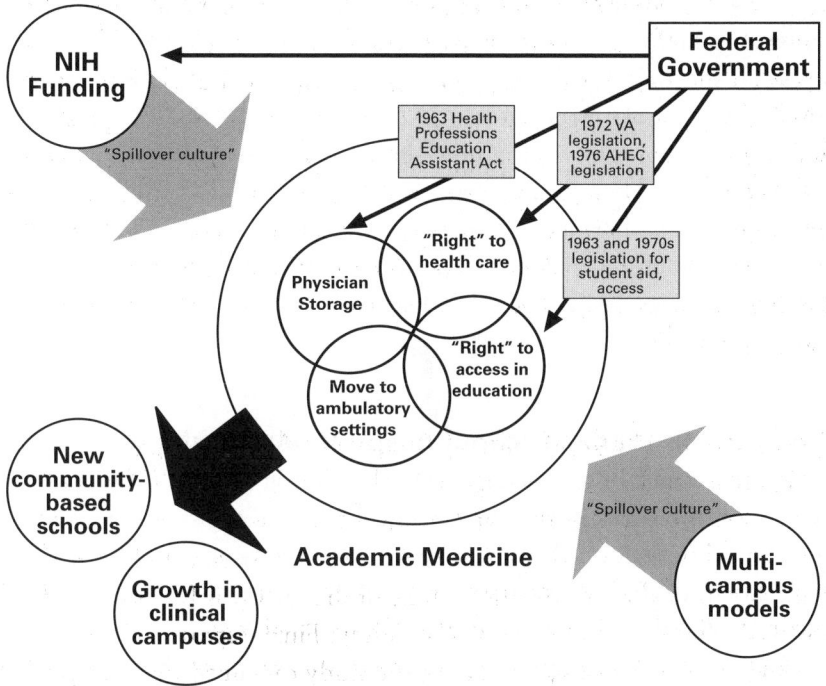

Figure 1

Historical Influences on the Development of Clinical Campuses

REVIEW OF THE RESEARCH LITERATURE

Scant scholarly attention has been paid to regional campuses at U.S. medical schools; we are aware of no peer-reviewed published literature that specifically addresses these organizational entities. Furthermore, there is no published history of the development of these campuses in the context of medical education in the United States. To provide a research context for this study, we reviewed the literature in four areas: community-based schools, medical school-teaching hospital relationships, branch campuses in higher education, and reports on clinical campuses.

Studies on community-based schools

The development of the so-called "community-based" schools and the origins of clinical campuses are inextricably linked. The new medical schools of the 1960s share many commonalities with regional campuses, especially those started in the 1970s. Several books (Bowers & Purcell, 1978; Hunt, 1979; Lippard & Purcell, 1972) chronicle the rationale and development of community-based schools. These books outline the strengths and weaknesses of the community-based model and underscore the importance of relationship building among medical school, hospital, and community—an important theme in the development and management of clinical campuses as well. For example, Aronson and Murray (1979) compared a specific clerkship experience in a community-based setting to that in a traditional tertiary hospital. They enumerated advantages for medical students at the community-based hospital—such as more intimate contact with attending physicians, greater self-reliance, and more significant responsibilities—but also disadvantages, such as lack of adequate library facilities, research, and student interaction.

Literature on medical school-hospital relationships

Because much of the management of a clinical campus is nurturing the relationship between the main medical school campus, on one hand, and a local hospital, on the other, we reviewed essays and studies on the management of clinical affiliations. One of the earliest is Keyes et al. (1977) "Medical School—Clinical Affiliation Study: Final Report." While not focusing on regional campuses *per se*, the study examined the management of medical school-teaching hospital relationships with the aim to identify good practices in effective partnerships. They found a "discernable trend… toward replacing department-to-hospital service affiliations with institution-wide, medical school-to-hospital agreements" (p. 124), a development that is reflected in several histories in the regional campuses in this current study. Keyes and colleagues also identified the importance of institutional history and self-image in the dynamics of the relationship. They stressed a number of good practices required of both hospital and medical school leaders to make the relationships effective.

Derzon's essay (1978) also addressed the alliances between medical school and hospital, although he, like Keyes, did not focus on clinical campuses specifically. Using a metaphor of marriage, Derzon suggested that healthy relationships depend on mutual success, bilateral leadership, ability to resolve conflicts, mutual understanding of education and business, and organizational alignment. Beljan (1979) also used the marriage analogy to describe the relationship between community hospitals and medical schools.

Literature on branch, satellite, and regional campuses in higher education

The "branch" campus model is not unique to medical education. Many colleges and universities maintain similar structures. We looked for parallel circumstances and lessons learned from these books and articles. Lee and Bowen (1971) traced the historical development of the multicampus university. More recent studies have focused on particular aspects of managing and governing branch campuses. Nickerson and Schaefer (2001) studied the characteristics of branch campus faculty. Dengerink (2001) posited a conceptual model of multiple identities in hybrid organization to understand the organization and culture of branch campuses. Other studies (Creswell, 1985; Deil & Barshis, 1996; Parkin, 1999; Smith, 1992; Watts, 1991) have concentrated on typology, governance, institutional identity, and collaboration in the satellite setting.

Reports and studies on clinical campuses

In an early description of the development of a regional campus, Costsonas, Getz, and Newman (1979) asserted a "territorial imperative" between main campus and regional campus, in which faculty at the main site questioned the quality of education at the distant site. They concluded, "we were all raised in a climate which prized independency, and now find ourselves in a climate in which the acceptance of our interdependence is both difficult and necessary for survival" (p. 71).

Several unpublished reports on clinical campuses have been conducted over the years. Watt et al. (1993) conducted an investigation on ten geographically separated campuses. They found that these sites produced value for the medical school and teaching hospital, increased the size and diversity of the patient base, posed extra recruiting challenges for faculty, appeared to have comparable student outcomes as the main campus, and presented management challenges in operations, governance, and faculty development. In another unpublished account, Swick (2000) detailed the history, organizational structure, faculty and student characteristics, and experiences of regional campuses at 31 U.S. medical schools.

The literature review revealed several gaps in the understanding of regional clinical campuses. First, despite one individual case study of the early development of a regional campus, no published national studies on the topic exist. Second, there is not a published thorough examination of the historical context of these entities. Watt et al. (1993) and Swick (2000) discuss historical rationales, but their evidence is based on a limited number of interviews and not on sources such as written documentation and published histories of medical education. Third, with some clinical campuses approaching their 30-year anniversaries and others just in the planning stages, there has not been an examination of the role of these entities in medical education at the beginning of the 21st century. This study aimed to address those gaps.

3. Methods

With the historical context and existing research in mind, we aimed to understand the organizational characteristics of, management relationships in, and student experiences at the nation's regional clinical campuses. This section details the methods we used to undertake the study.

Research Questions

We were interested in addressing the following questions:

1. What are the organizational characteristics of the clinical campus (e.g., year of founding, number of students and faculty, faculty appointment and promotion policies, types of educational experiences, sources of funding, type and size of clinical facilities)?
2. Why were clinical campuses founded and maintained?
3. What are the educational experiences of students at clinical campuses?
4. How do administrators perceive the organizational, management and governance relationships of the clinical campus and main campus?

The first research question was a broad survey question intended for the entire population of regional sites. The next three questions were focused on a smaller sample of campuses to be answered through in-depth site visits and document analysis.

Research Design

The research questions demanded multiple methods. Our first question was a descriptive inquiry on the status of clinical campuses in U.S. medical education. We designed two survey instruments for this purpose. Our next three questions called for a qualitative inquiry because we wanted to understand the context and structure of clinical campuses. In this type of research, Merriam (1998) says, researchers "seek to discover and understand a phenomenon, a process, or the perspectives and worldviews of the people involved" (p. 11).

Research Methods

The research methods involved several stages. This section reports on the process for each part.

Determining the Site Visit Population

Based on previous research (Swick, 2000; Watt et al., 1993) and LCME definitions, we constructed a list of campuses that met various classifications (see appendix 2). Because of differences in data gathering, reporting, and definitions, there were inconsistencies in whether a particular campus met the threshold of a regional campus. For example, Watt et al. (1993) did not include the Knoxville and Chattanooga campuses of the University of Tennessee College of Medicine but the LCME did.

For these reasons, we devised our own criteria of a "regional clinical campus." Our primary objective at this stage was *not* to identify the entire population of clinical campuses but rather to ascertain those that were substantial in scope and operations and, thus, adequate for site visits. We purposefully excluded community-based schools at this point because we wanted to examine, among other things, the relationship between the main academic medical center and the distant site. Community-based schools, by definition, do not have a main academic medical center. We sent an email query to the associate deans for medical education at all 125 U.S. allopathic medical schools. From the responses, we identified 31 regional sites associated with traditional (i.e. non-community based) schools for further inquiry.

Survey to Medical Education Deans

We sent a detailed survey to the associate dean for medical education at 23 medical schools that operated these 31 campuses (see appendix 3). All the surveys were returned. The survey asked about reporting relationships of the regional dean, the year the campus was founded, the number of clerkships offered, the percentage of students who attend the campus for the full-year, and the amount of funding transferred to the regional campus for medical student education. From these responses, we determined that five sites did not fit our definition. We narrowed the remaining 26 to a group of ten for site visits (see appendix 4). In selecting the sites, we wanted to insure that we included a representation of campuses around the country, public and private in control, and older and newer sites. While eight of the ten clinical campuses enroll third-year students for the whole year, we intentionally included two with variations. The University of California San Francisco, Fresno has a six-month program as well as a rotational program. The University of Florida College of Medicine requires all third-year medical students to attend its Jacksonville campus from two to 24 weeks, with an average of 12 weeks, although none attends for the full year. A list of the ten schools can be found in appendix 5.

Site Visits

We contacted each regional dean about our proposed site visit. All agreed to participate. Two members of our four-member research team attended each site visit, conducted between February and May 2002. To insure consistency, one team member attended all ten. We devised a standard interview schedule and protocol (see appendix 6). We requested to meet with a defined group of representatives, including the regional dean, hospital CEO or designee, president of the elected medical staff, two clerkship directors, a group of third-year medical students, and a group of faculty members. Each regional dean identified the specific interviewees at each site. Except for a few variations, we met with similar representatives on all ten campuses.

We conducted interviews using a focused interview approach, which employs a set of structured, open-ended questions (Yin, 1994). We used an interview guide (see appendix 7) to structure the interview, but the study design allowed us to probe additional issues and concerns raised by each respondent. At each site, we interviewed between 5 and 15 individuals and between 5 and 17 participants took part in focus groups. Each interview lasted between one-half to one and a half hours. In total, over 225 people were included in the on-site portion of this study.

Prior to the start of each interview or focus group, we explained the purpose and goals of the study. We discussed confidentiality issues, explaining to participants that they would not be quoted by name or with institutional identifiers in this or any subsequent reports. For this reason, throughout this report we distinguish the source of quotations only by generic position (e.g. faculty member, hospital administrator) and not with institutional identifiers.

Since qualitative methodologists are impartial toward audio recording versus hand recording (Yin [1994] states the method is a matter of personal preference), one researcher hand recorded notes of each conversation.

Interviews with Medical School Deans

While our primary unit of analysis was the regional campus, we also wanted to obtain data from the main medical school deans about their perspectives of the clinical site. The deans of the University of Arizona and University of Oklahoma were present at the clinical campus during our visits, so we interviewed them on-site. We conducted phone interviews with four additional deans.

Written Documentation

We requested written document from each campus prior to the visit to help us understand the current and historical context of the clinical campus. While the specific types of written material varied by campus, we received items such as:

- Student "marketing" materials (i.e., information distributed to first- and second-year medical students explaining the facilities, services, and operations of the regional campus)
- Student policies/handbook specific to the regional campus
- Strategic planning documents
- Documents/materials about why the regional campus was created
- Financial statement
- Portions of LCME self-study reports
- Other relevant information

Each campus provided at least 100 pages of information, some many times that amount.

Survey of the Known Population of Clinical Campuses

Based on the experiences at the ten regional campuses, we wrote a second questionnaire to send to the regional deans of all clinical campuses that were known to us (see survey instrument in Appendix 8). At this stage, we wanted to survey the entire population of regional clinical campuses, *including* those at community-based schools. Using previous studies and the review of literature, we identified 41 regional campuses to include in the survey population.[1] Thirty-nine of the 41 completed the questionnaire (95 percent response rate).[2] The data from these survey responses, coupled with the in-depth data gathered during the ten site visits, produced a comprehensive database on the institutional and organizational characteristics of the population of clinical campuses in the United States. (See appendix 9 for schools included and excluded from our list.)

Data Analysis

Site Visits

At the conclusion of each visit, a researcher transcribed site notes into word processing software. Then, upon completion of all ten site visits, each member of the research team reviewed the written transcripts of all visits. Each team member developed schemata of themes and "recurring regularities" (Guba, 1978) that emerged from the data. The team met to analyze our individual themes and to develop meta-themes, which guided the description and analysis in this report.

Surveys

The results of both surveys were entered into Excel database for data storage and analyses. We examined and rank-ordered responses for each question, and used the results to guide our descriptive analysis of the regional campus structure and organization.

Limitations

Like all research, this study had limitations that arose from our methodological choices. The main findings, reported in sections 5 through 7, are based on qualitative interviews during site visits at ten regional clinical campuses. Because we included 40 percent of the clinical campuses at traditional medical schools in our study sample, the generalizability of the

---

[1] The total population is 42 clinical campuses. At the time of our inquiry, however, the University of Nevada School of Medicine was undergoing organizational restructuring so it was unclear which of its campuses—Reno or Las Vegas—was considered its main campus and which was considered its clinical campus. Therefore, we excluded it from further analyses.

[2] Two schools did not return the survey: Michigan State University–Saginaw did not for unknown reasons; and the University of Illinois Chicago College of Medicine–Urbana Champaign did not consider itself only a clinical campus because it also offers basic science instruction.

findings increases and we can offer richer descriptions and more powerful explanations (Miles and Huberman, 1994). Nevertheless, the findings may not be predictive to the entire population of clinical campuses of traditional (non-community based) medical schools. Furthermore, because we did not include community-based school campuses in the site visit population, the findings in sections 5 through 7 may not be generalizable to that population. We leave those decisions up to the reader; whether this study's findings apply to other institutions is up to the people in those institutions (Merriam, 1998).

Our research focused on the clinical campus as the unit of analysis. Regional campus interviewees relied on their perceptions of the relationship with the main campus. It is these perceptions that we found interesting and which are reported in detail in sections 6 and 7. A majority of the main campus deans were also interviewed; their perceptions typically matched those leaders at the regional site. It is worth emphasizing, though, that faculty and students at the main campuses were not included in the data collection process. This was outside the scope of our study.

4. AN OVERVIEW OF THE CLINICAL BRANCH CAMPUSES AT U.S. MEDICAL SCHOOLS

The regional branch campuses of U.S. medical schools reflect the organizational and administrative complexities of their parent campuses. These regional campuses vary considerably in the breadth of their operations and organizational structure. This section reviews the organizational characteristics of all clinical campuses—those affiliated both with traditional medical schools and with community-based schools—on aspects such as founding date, size and characteristics of faculty, nature of the administrative and educational infrastructure, and types of student education programs. As noted in the methods section, we surveyed the regional deans of 41 clinical campuses. Thirty-nine of the surveys were completed.

Year of Founding

The majority (62 percent) of clinical branch campuses were founded during the first-half of the 1970s, consistent with the ethos of the times to increase access to health care and to academic medical centers in many communities (see Table 1). During the late 1970s and 1980s, relatively few branch campuses were started, but in the 1990s, another nine campuses (23 percent) began. These more recent additions came as patient care moved to ambulatory settings and some academic medical centers searched for new clinical opportunities for their medical students.

Table 1

Dates of Founding of Regional Clinical Campuses at U.S. Medical Schools (n=39)

Years	Number of Regional Clinical Campuses Founded
1970-1975	24
1976-1980	2
1981-1985	1
1986-1990	3
1991-1995	5
1996-2000	4

Table 2
Other Health-Related Programs of the University Offered at the Regional Campus (n=23)

Regional Campus	Nursing	Pharmacy	Physician Assistant	Allied Health	Public Health	Dentistry	Other
Drexel-Alleghany General Hospital (Pittsburgh)			x				EMS
Drexel-Monmouth Medical Center (Long Branch, NJ)				x		x	lab tech
Michigan State-Grand Rapids	x	x	x				physician therapy, occup. therapy
Michigan State-Kalamazoo		x	x				
Penn State-York		x	x	x		x	pastoral care
Texas Tech-Amarillo		x		x			
Texas Tech-El Paso		x					
Texas Tech-Odessa	x		x	x			
Univ. of Alabama-Tuscaloosa	x						health education, psychology, CSD
Univ. of Arizona-Phoenix	x	x			x		
Univ. of Florida-Jacksonville	x	x				x	
Univ. of Illinois-Peoria	x				x		
Univ. of Illinois-Rockford	x	x			x		
Univ. of Kansas-Wichita					x		
Univ. of North Dakota Northwest Campus	x		x				
Univ. of Oklahoma-Tulsa	x	x		x	x		
Univ. of South Dakota West River	x						
Univ. of South Dakota Yankton	x	x	x				
Univ. of Tennessee Chattanooga	x	x		x			
Univ. of Tennessee-Knoxville		x				x	oral maxillofacial surgery
Univ. of Texas Medical Branch-Austin	x	x					
Univ. of Wisconsin-Western Campus (LaCrosse)	x	x	x	x			nuclear med., clin. microbiology, radiation therapy
West Virginia Univ-Charleston	x	x				x	social work

No Additional Schools Reported (n=16)

Mercer-Memorial Health University Medical Center (Savannah), Michigan State University-Flint, Michigan State University-Upper Peninsula, Penn State-Lehigh Valley, SUNY Upstate-Binghamton, Temple-West Penn Hospital (Pittsburgh), Tufts-Baystate Medical Center (Springfield), UMDNJ/RWJ-Camden, University of Alabama-Huntsville, UCSF-Fresno, University of Iowa-Des Moines, University of North Dakota-Fargo, University of North Dakota-Southwest Campus, University of South Carolina-Greenville, University of Virginia-Roanoke, University of Wisconsin-Milwaukee

Administrative Structure

We were interested in the scope of administrative infrastructure at the regional sites. We posed three questions to provide an indication of the variation among sites. First, do other health-related schools or colleges of the university offer programs at the regional campus? Second, how many administrative personnel, other than the regional dean, are employed by the medical school at the regional campus? Third, from what sources is the regional dean's salary supported?

Many of the regional campuses offer other health-related programs in addition to medical education (see Table 2). Of those responding to this question, 16 campuses offer nursing programs, 16 offer pharmacy, 8 offer physician assistant programs, 7 offer allied health, 5 offer public health, 5 offer dentistry, and 8 offer other types of programs. In total, 23 of the responding schools provide health-related educational programs in addition to medical education; 16 only teach medical students.

Table 3
Number of Administrative Personnel (FTE) Employed by the Medical School at the Regional Campus
(n=38)

Administrative Personnel FTE	Regional Campus	Administrative Personnel FTE	Regional Campus
0.0	Drexel-Monmouth	3.0	South Dakota-Yankton
0.0	MSU-Kalamazoo	4.0	Texas Tech-Amarillo
0.0	MSU-Upper Peninsula	4.5	North Dakota-Southwest
0.0	Penn State-Lehigh Valley	4.75	Tennessee-Chattanooga
0.0	Penn State-New York	5.0	Illinois-Rockford
0.0	South Carolina-Greenville	5.2	West Virginia-Charleston
0.0	Tufts-Baystate	8.0	UMDNJ/RWJ-Camden
0.0	UTMB-Austin	8.0	Alabama-Tuscaloosa
0.0	Wisconsin-LaCrosse	8.0	Oklahoma-Tulsa
0.3	Virginia-Roanoke	17.0	SUNY Upstate-Binghamton
1.0	North Dakota-Northwest	19.0	Florida-Jacksonville
1.0	South Dakota-West River	20.0	Tennessee-Knoxville
1.2	Temple-West Penn Hospital	21.0	Arizona-Phoenix
1.5	Iowa-Des Moines	21.2	Alabama-Huntsville
1.8	MSU-Grand Rapids	23.0	MSU-Flint
2.0	Wisconsin-Milwaukee	64.0	Texas Tech-El Paso
2.2	North Dakota-Fargo	71.0	UCSF-Fresno
2.5	Drexel-Allegheny	100.0	Texas Tech-Odessa
3.0	Mercer-Savannah	131.17	Kansas-Wichita

MODE = 0.0   MEDIAN = 3.0

Most regional campuses rely on a small administrative infrastructure. The median administrative personnel full-time equivalency employed by the medical school (excluding the regional dean if he/she is a school employee) is 3.0 (see Table 3). The mode (most common response) is zero; nine of the 39 schools responding to this question have no medical school employees at the regional site. Another 19 sites have ten or fewer FTE positions.

Sources of Regional Dean's Salary

There is considerable variation in who provides the salary support for the regional dean. As noted in Figure 2, the medical school pays the whole salary for 13 regional deans. At eight campuses, the regional dean's salary is paid entirely (or almost entirely) by the hospital. At another seven, the salary of the regional dean is split evenly (or nearly evenly). These data, coupled with the number of administrative personnel, are suggestive of the different administrative arrangements medical schools have constructed for their geographically separate medical education programs. Some schools have

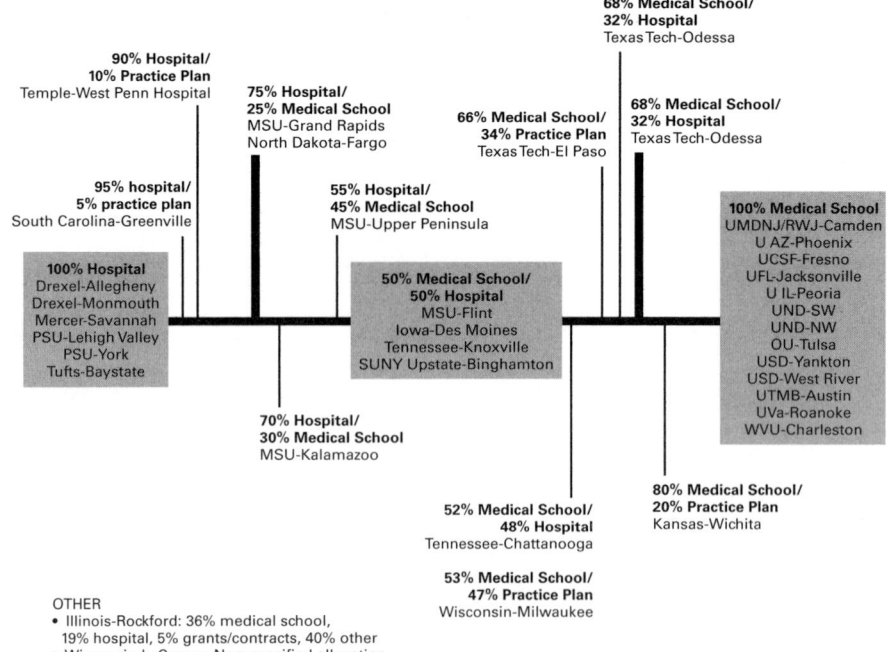

Figure 2

Sources of Support for Regional Dean's Salary

Table 4
Regional Clinical Campuses Whose Faculty are NIH Grant Recipients (n=39)

Number of Faculty with NIH Grants	Number of Campuses
0	23
1	4
2	3
3	4
4	2
5	1
6	0
7	1
8	0
9	0
10+	1

developed an "ownership" model—employing a sizable staff, operating their own buildings, and treating the regional dean as a full-time employee of the medical school. Others have adopted a "contractor" model, in which they outsource the regional program to a hospital, medical center, or regional consortium. Under this arrangement, the regional dean is a full-time hospital employee, few or no university employees work at the regional site, and the university doesn't have a separate building or physical presence. Other regional campuses are a hybrid of these two extremes.

The Research Enterprise of Regional Campuses

Regional campuses primarily focus on the educational and clinical missions of the medical school. Not surprisingly, they have small research enterprises. Twenty-nine of 39 respondents (74 percent) indicated they receive less than $2.5 million in external research funding annually from all sources. Two campuses reported annual funding between $2.5 - $5 million; three receive between $5-10 million, and three receive more than $10 million on an annual basis.

NIH grant funding is a common benchmark of the research intensity of a campus. Few faculty members at regional campuses are the recipients of NIH grants. As Table 4 indicates, the vast majority of clinical campuses do not have any faculty members with NIH funding.

Table 5
Institutional Sponsor of Residency Programs Offered at the Clinical Campus (n=35)

Institutional Sponsor of Residency Programs	Number of Respondents
Hospital or regional consortium	20
The medical school, with the same ACGME institutional sponsor number as the main medical school campus	2
The medical school, with a different ACGME institutional sponsor number as the main medical school campus	12
Both hospital and medical school	1

Medical Education

Regional campuses sponsor medical education programs for both residents and medical students. All but two regional campuses offer residency programs. As indicated in Table 5, most of these residencies are freestanding programs sponsored by the hospital or hospital-consortia. A smaller number are sponsored by the medical school—separate from those sponsored at the main campus. Only two regional campuses offer residency programs with the same ACGME institutional sponsor number as the main medical school campus.

Regional campuses can accommodate third-year medical students under two primary arrangements. Students either attend for the whole year or they rotate in and out for specific clerkships. Several permutations, however, exist within these two models. Some medical schools allow students to attend the regional campus for the full year but also permit other students to rotate for specific clerkships if space permits. Others enable students to attend less than full-year but longer than one or two clerkships. As illustrated in Table 6, 26 schools have some portion of their third-year class attend for the full-year.

Many models also exist for assigning students to the regional campus. The most common mechanism is to let students decide if they want to attend. Eighteen campuses use this voluntary method, most with the caveat that an assignment or lottery system can be used if too few or too many students volunteer. Three campuses use a lottery system. Four require students to indicate a preference during the application process and then assign students based on that preference. One program (MSU, Upper Peninsula) has an interview and application process for its spots. One campus reported using a combination of several methods.

Table 6
Percentage of Third-year Medical School Class that Attends the Regional Campus for the Whole Year
(n=26)

Regional Campus at which third-year students enroll for the full year	Percentage of third-year class that attends regional campus for the whole year	Can other students rotate for specific clerkships?
Drexel-Alleghany General Hospital (Pittsburgh)	10%	yes
Drexel-Monmouth Medical Center (Long Branch, NJ)	1%	yes
Mercer-Memorial Health University Medical Center	25-30%	no
Michigan State University-Flint	19%	no
Michigan State University-Grand Rapids	25-27%	no
Michigan State University-Upper Peninsula	8%	no
SUNY Upstate-Binghamton	25%	no
Temple-West Penn Hospital (Pittsburgh)	16%	yes
Texas Tech-Amarillo	34%	no
Texas Tech-El Paso	44%	no
Tufts-Baystate Medical Center (Springfield)	15%	yes
UMDNJ/RWJ-Camden	33%	no
Univ. of Alabama-Huntville	12-15%	yes
Univ. of Alabama-Tuscaloosa	12-15%	yes
Univ. of Arizona-Phoenix	30-40%	yes
Univ. of Illinois-Peoria	17%	no
Univ. of Illinois-Rockford	17%	no
Univ. of Kansas-Wichita	30%	no
Univ. of North Dakota Southwest Campus	40%	yes
Univ. of Oklahoma-Tulsa	16-20%	no
Univ. of South Carolina-Greenville	20%	no
Univ. of South Dakota-West River	25%	no
Univ. of South Dakota-Yankton	24%	no
Univ. of Tennessee-Knoxville	5%	yes
Univ. of Texas Medical Branch-Austin	5%	yes
West Virginia Univ-Charleston	30%	no

No third-year students attend for the full year
(n = 11)

Penn State-Lehigh Valley Medical Center, Penn State-York, Texas Tech-Odessa, UCSF-Fresno, University of Florida-Jacksonville, University of Iowa-Des Moines, University of North Dakota-Northwest Campus, University of Tennessee-Chattanooga, University of Virginia-Roanoke, University of Wisconsin-Milwaukee, University of Wisconsin-Western Campus (LaCrosse)

Faculty at the Regional Campuses

Most of the regional campuses that responded to our survey rely heavily on volunteer in additional to full-time faculty. The results are consistent with other research that has demonstrated the importance of volunteer faculty for the delivery of the medical education program, particularly in ambulatory settings (Fields et al., 1998; Jones & Sanderson, 1996). As noted in Table 7, the majority of regional campuses do not offer tenure or tenure-track appointments. Of those with full-time faculty, 13 of the 31 branch campuses do not have any tenured or tenure-track faculty. These findings also are comparable to national data on faculty appointments for clinical faculty members.

One measure of traditional faculty roles and responsibilities is the level of involvement in institutional governance, i.e., a role in curriculum, admissions, student progress, and promotion and tenure decisions. We were interested whether faculty at regional campuses were involved in these activities. In fact, the vast majority of regional campuses have faculty representation on major committees at the main campus: promotion and tenure, curriculum, admission, and student progress. Table 8 displays this committee representation.

It is worth noting that the absence of committee representation does not necessarily mean that the regional campus faculty is excluded from institutional decision-making processes. One campus, for example, indicated that regional faculty have the opportunity to be involved on all committees but were only participating in two because of constraints of time and distance.

The coin of the realm in self-governance for faculty is their involvement in promotion and tenure decisions. We asked about the presence of a local promotions committee as one measure, albeit a crude and inexact one, for faculty self-governance at the local level. The vast majority of regional campuses (27 of 38 respondents) do not have local tenure and promotions committees. Again, the absence of this local committee does not necessarily mean that branch campus faculty are excluded from decision-making or don't benefit from traditional faculty prerogatives or roles.

> **Regional campuses with their own promotion and tenure committee, separate from the main campus:** UMDNJ/RWJ-Camden (department level), University of Alabama-Huntsville, University of Alabama-Tuscaloosa, University of Arizona-Phoenix, UCSF-Fresno, University of Illinois-Peoria, University of Illinois-Rockford, University of Kansas-Wichita, University of South Carolina-Greenville, University of Tennessee-Chattanooga, University of Tennessee-Knoxville

Table 7
Number of Full-time, Part-time, and Volunteer Faculty at Regional Campuses (n=38)

Regional Campus	Full-Time Faculty	Percent tenured or tenure-eligible	Percent non-tenure track	Part-Time Faculty	Voluntary Faculty
Drexel-Allegheny General Hospital (Pittsburgh)	78	0%	100%	114	
Drexel-Monmouth Medical Center (Long Branch, NJ)	0	--	--	0	145
Mercer-Memorial Health University Medical Center	50	2%	98%	0	50
Michigan State-Flint	64	0%	100%	0	446
Michigan State-Grand Rapids	2	100%	0%	58	875
Michigan State-Kalamazoo	50	0%	100%	18	500
Michigan State-Upper Peninsula	0	--	--	8	182
Penn State-Lehigh Valley Medical Center (Allentown)	0	--	--	0	425
Penn State-York	15	0%	100%	0	15
SUNY Upstate-Binghamton	6	17%	83%	120-130	300
Temple-West Penn Hospital (Pittsburgh)	0	--	--	0	120
Texas Tech-Amarillo	64*	14%	86%	10	75
Texas Tech-El Paso	151*	15%	85%	--	--
Texas Tech-Odessa	48	0%	100%	5	0
Tufts-Baystate	250	0%	100%	10	750
UMDNJ/RWJ-Camden	270	0%	100%	4	118
University of Alabama-Huntsville	23	57%	43%	5	294
University of Alabama-Tuscaloosa	28	39%	61%	4	260
University of Arizona-Phoenix	8	25%	75%	22	350
University of Calif. San Francisco-Fresno	85	5%	85%	40	400
University of Florida-Jacksonville	259	41%	59%	15	163
University of Illinois-Peoria	95*	22%	78%	60	700+
University of Illinois-Rockford (1)	119*	13%	87%	130	450
University of Iowa-Des Moines	20	0%	100%	100	100
University of Kansas-Wichita (2)	43*	67%	33%	59	778
University of North Dakota-Northwest Campus	0	--	--	3	79
University of North Dakota-Southwest Campus	0	--	--	7	200
University of Oklahoma-Tulsa	75*	29%	71%	33	847
University of South Carolina-Greenville	120	0%	100%		100
University of South Dakota-West River	0	--	--	8	150
University of South Dakota-Yankton	2	100%	0%	48	--
University of Tennessee-Chattanooga	83	8%	92%	34	257
University of Tennessee-Knoxville	210*	30%	70%	50	80
University of Texas Medical Branch-Austin	20	0%	100%	50	--
University of Virginia-Roanoke	75	0%	100%	3	100
University of Wisconsin-Milwaukee (3)	55	0%	100%	0	195
University of Wisconsin-Western Campus (LaCrosse)	88	0%	100%	--	--
West Virgina University-Charleston	73	22%	78%	3	100+

(1) plus 15 FT in "other" track
(2) plus 8 FT in "other" track
(3) plus 36 FT in "other" track

* = Respondent discrepancy. School's response for (number of full-time tenured or tenure-eligible faculty + number of full-time non-tenure-track faculty + number of full-time other track faculty) does not match school's response for number of total full-time faculty. In these cases, we reported the sum of the subcategories.

Table 8
Representation of Regional Campus Faculty Members on School-wide Committees at the Main Medical School Campus
(n=31)

Regional Campus	Curriculum	Admissions	Student Progress/Review	Promotion
Drexel-Allegheny General Hospital (Pittsburgh)	x	x		x
Drexel-Monmouth Medical Center (Long Branch, NJ)	x			x
Mercer-Memorial Health University Medical Center	x			x
Michigan State University-Flint	x	x	x	x
Michigan State-Grand Rapids			x	
Michigan State-Kalamazoo	x	x	x	
SUNY Upstate-Binghamton	x	x	x	x
Temple-West Penn Hospital (Pittsburgh)	x	x	x	
Texas Tech-Amarillo	x	x	x	x
Texas Tech-El Paso	x	x	x	x
Texas Tech-Odessa				x
Tufts-Baystate	x	x	x	x
UMDNJ/RWJ-Camden	x	x	x	x
University of Alabama-Huntsville	x	x	x	x
University of Alabama-Tuscaloosa	x	x	x	
University of Arizona-Phoenix	x	x	x	
UCSF-Fresno	x		x	x
University of Florida-Jacksonville	x	x	x	x
University of Illinois-Peoria	x	x	x	x
University of Illinois-Rockford	x	x	x	x
University of Kansas-Wichita	x	x	x	x
University of North Dakota-Northwest Campus	x		x	
University of North Dakota-Southwest Campus	x	x	x	x
University of Oklahoma-Tulsa	x	x	x	x
University of South Dakota-Yankton		x		
University of Tennessee-Chattanooga	x	x		x
University of Tennessee-Knoxville		x	x	x
University of Virginia-Roanoke			x	
University of Wisconsin-Milwaukee	x	x	x	x
University of Wisconsin-Western Campus (LaCrosse)	x	x	x	x
West Virgina University-Charleston	x	x	x	x
Total number of campuses with faculty representation on each committee:	26	24	25	23

No regional faculty representation on main medical school committees
(n = 7)
Michigan State University-Upper Peninsula, Penn State-Lehigh Valley Medical Center (Allentown), Penn State-York, University of Iowa-Des Moines, University of South Carolina-Greenville, University of South Dakota-West River, University of Texas Medical Branch-Austin

5. WHY A REGIONAL CLINICAL CAMPUS?

With the broad organizational characteristics defined for all clinical campuses, we now turn to an analysis and discussion of findings from the ten site visits. The remaining sections in this report focus on those ten campuses.

Our second research question investigated the reasons why the regional campuses were founded. The reasons for the regional clinical campus vary by source. The medical school, the primary hospitals at the regional site, and the local community had different motivations for establishing and maintaining a branch campus. Our interviews and document analysis of the ten campuses suggest the following rationales.

Benefits to the Medical School

As noted in our review of the history of these campuses, medical schools developed branch campuses, especially in the 1970s, to counteract the impending physician shortage in their states and in certain communities. Some medical school leaders in our study noted that the branch campuses allow them to focus on primary care and community settings in ways that the main campus could not by itself. For example, the programs at UCSF-Fresno, Alabama-Huntsville, SUNY Upstate-Binghamton, and WVU-Charleston provide a venue to specifically focus on primary care. In fact, the Huntsville campus was for a time called the School of Primary Medical Care. For research-intensive medical schools such at San Francisco and Alabama, the regional campus offers a different type of educational experience—more clinically focused—that, as one Fresno clerkship director noted, "enriches the educational product."

Another benefit of the regional campus for the main medical school is a larger patient base. Many of the schools in our study have limitations in their main location. Several are located small cities: Mercer (Macon), Florida (Gainesville), Arizona (Tucson), West Virginia (Morgantown). The regional sites are in larger, fast-growing population centers that provide crucial patient volumes: Savannah, Jacksonville, Phoenix, and Charleston. Two other schools—Robert Wood Johnson Medical School and Tufts University—are located in densely populated areas but the regional campuses offer the same benefits. For this reason, the regional sites recognize their importance to the main campus. One faculty member said, "[The main campus] couldn't do the whole third and fourth years without us. They couldn't reabsorb all the students." A regional administrator noted, "We have been able to support 40 students each year. That is a recognized value to them."

A third benefit to the main campus is the broadened political network offered by a presence in an additional locale. For public medical schools that depend on good relations with state legislators, the additional campus expands that support. Officials at Arizona, Florida, Oklahoma, SUNY Upstate, UCSF, and West Virginia all mentioned how the branch campus created new allies in the state government. For some schools, the regional campus served as a political buffer against the development of another medical school in the city. The Phoenix campus of the University of Arizona is a prime example.

Benefits to the Hospital

Leaders at the hospitals affiliated with the regional campus expressed numerous benefits for hosting a regional medical education program. The most-often cited was that the affiliation enhanced the hospital's standing as an academic medical center, part of its overall mission. One hospital leader said, "It is part of the very essence of who and what we are. Without the relationship, [the hospital] would just as soon go away." Another agreed: "Why have students? It's our mission. If you take away students and the underserved, then I don't have an institution." Still another hospital leader noted that the relationship enhanced the hospital's academic image, offering strategic benefits such as improved ability to capture state funds for research.

Hospitals benefited in their marketing initiatives. Several of the hospitals added "university" to their name when the clinical campus started. The CEO of Baystate Medical Center said, "There is marquee value being known as 'the Western Campus' of Tufts. It enhances the visibility and prestige of the hospital." Memorial Health University Hospital wanted to be viewed among Savannah's community of retirees as "Georgia's equivalent of the major teaching hospital you loved back East."

A third benefit to hospitals is in recruitment of residents and faculty members. One of the hospital directors in Phoenix expressed a common sentiment: "That's what gets the faculty and physicians to come to a place like this. Medical students add to the recruitment." Several hospitals viewed the medical student education program as a feeder system into their residency programs (although they also noted that idea typically fell short of its goal.)

A corollary advantage to high-quality faculty recruitment is an improvement in the quality of care. High-quality faculty and high-quality residents make for a better hospital, the thinking goes. In some cases, the affiliation also expanded the medical center's clinical research program, also adding to the quality of care. In turn, hospitals have used the relationship to convey its "quality of care" message to its market. As one executive noted, "The hospital uses its relationship with the medical school to promote the quality of care to the community. The logo of the university is on the printing materials for the hospital."

Despite the varied benefits asserted by leaders of the affiliated hospitals, they also noted that the medical education program was primarily about residents, not students. "Students are the chrome bumpers," said one hospital official. "They come with the GME program." Another admitted, "My primary obligation is to the resident program, not to medical students." A third colleague stated, "The residencies are what this is about. The medical students are part of that package."

Benefits to the Local Community

The regional campus brings advantages to the community in which it is located. Consistent with the historical reasons for the development of these campuses, the local community enjoys the benefits of increased physician supply. At many of the campuses we visited—Binghamton, Fresno, Huntsville, Jacksonville, and Tulsa, to name several—significant percentages of local doctors were educated at the clinical site. In fact, 50 percent of the residents in the Fresno program remain in the area to practice medicine, presumably meeting one of the original goals of the California legislature when it approved the campus in 1974.

The medical education program in the community also helps attract specialty physicians that the region might otherwise have difficulty recruiting. This is especially true in rural sites like Fresno. One community doctor emphasized, "The whole valley benefits from having providers attracted to this area.... A good example is surgery. Without the affiliation, the high-end academic center, it would be hard to attract them."

The regional campus also offers other benefits to the local community, similar to any community with an academic medical center: improved quality of care, increased opportunities for economic development, high levels of community service in health care because of student and faculty involvement, and enhanced prestige of the community.

6. MEDICAL STUDENT EDUCATION AT THE REGIONAL CAMPUS

THE EDUCATIONAL EXPERIENCE

One of the unanticipated observations by the co-directors of the AAMC Project on the Clinical Education of Medical Students was medical students' overwhelmingly positive reaction to their clinical educational experiences at regional clinical campuses. The Project, however, was not designed to further investigate this phenomenon. The current study aimed to understand medical students' educational experiences at regional campuses and the reasons for those experiences.

As noted in the methods section, we met with a group of third-year (and in some cases, fourth-year) medical students at each site who spent the entire third-year at the clinical campus (except in two cases: at UCSF Fresno, we met with Model Fresno participants, who spend six months at the regional campus. At the Jacksonville campus of the University of Florida College of Medicine, all students attend for two to 24 weeks.) We also met with the regional deans, at least two clerkship directors at each site, and a group of clinical faculty members.

Benefits

In every site visit, the students were positive and enthusiastic about the clinical experiences they had at the regional site. Regional deans were proud of that track record. One dean who spent time working at both campus settings said, "Students are delighted with their clinical experiences here. You don't always hear that [at the main campus]." Similar to Nutter and Whitcomb's findings (2001), the clerkship directors with whom we met were "highly motivated, enthusiastic, and committed to overcoming the challenges they faced" (p. 7). Faculty and students voiced many benefits to the clinical education experience at the regional site, which can be distilled into five distinct themes.

1. Regional Clinical Campuses are a Place for Educational Innovation

Regional faculty and administrators were passionate and confident about the role of the regional campus as an incubator for new educational ideas and practices. Each of the following comments comes from a different regional campus:

- "This is a site for pilot testing. We were the pilot site for a palliative care experience, which now will be introduced to [the main campus]. Our clerkship directors are more willing to give up some time. We currently have two pilot projects: (1) six one-half day seminars on a variety of interdisciplinary topics (geriatrics, evidence-based medicine, etc.) and (2) a continuity-of-care clinic. Our small size makes these projects more doable. A clinical campus like this is a primary place for innovation." (Assistant dean)

- "There have been several cases of the tail wagging the dog with medical student education innovations. For example, the bioethics center was started at [the regional campus].... This is a place for pilot testing, innovation, and change. We are an incubator." (Faculty member)

- "The clinical campus' critical mission is undergraduate medical education; that's not as high on the main campus. So, we can bring innovation with much more rigor and zeal.... We can be more innovative and creative.... As an educational program, we're not invested in a clinical delivery structure. We have flexibility because we're not tied to a particular facility or system." (Regional dean)

- "We brought up the IT component in the clerkship (PDAs, internet access, etc.). They have now replicated that [at the main campus]." (Clerkship director)

- "At our campus, faculty, students, and staff are enthusiastic and are ready for innovations, which is usually the strength of a clinical campus. The size of the campus allows innovations to take place. Faculty and staff listen to students. The culture here is that everyone works together to make this a better place." (Regional dean)

As these quotations suggest, the regional campus communities expressed several reasons for their ability to be innovative in the delivery of clinical education. First, regional campuses' smaller size facilitated development of new ideas. Second, these campuses claimed their *raison d'etre* was undergraduate medical education. Faculty were highly committed to this primary mission. Third, with fewer infrastructure and administrative layers, the campuses were less bureaucratic and could change more quickly. Fourth, medical education at the regional campus was more centralized, allowing curricular change to occur more easily. These experiences are in contrast to the findings of Nutter and Whitcomb (2001) who found:

> Traditionally, the responsibility for the design and conduct of the clerkships has been delegated almost entirely to the individual clinical departments. This situation is responsible to a great extent for the difficulty that schools have experienced in attempting to reform the clinical curriculum, particularly in integrating content across clerkships, and to improving teaching methods. (p. 7)

Despite their self-perception as incubators for innovation, regional campuses acknowledged difficulty in expanding this role. Innovations "have to be done in the corner," reported one regional dean, because of concern about LCME requirements for comparable clerkship experiences. This fear frustrated some regional campus deans and faculty, who believed that this requirement was unrealistic. For example, a clerkship director said, "We've endeavored to be separate but equal, but the experiences in the clerkship are different." These reactions are similar to findings in the Nutter and Whitcomb report, which found that medical schools have difficulty "ensur[ing] to a reasonable degree that during a single clerkship all students are having comparable educational experiences. In fact, many schools recognize that this is not the case" (p. 6).

2. Regional Campuses Offers Small, Personal Learning Environments
The litany of benefits that students and faculty offered for the regional campus is like those found in the undergraduate admissions literature on the differences between a small liberal arts college and a large research university. One of the most frequently marshaled advantages was small size. Fewer students, fewer residents, and few or no fellows allow closer interaction between medical students and attending physicians and between medical students and patients. As a result, students developed strong relationships with faculty and staff (both student services staff and well as nurses, etc.), benefited from one-on-one lectures, had numerous opportunities for meaningful interactions with their fellow students, and received significant hands-on training. The organizations tend to be less hierarchical and "less ivory tower."

3. Regional Campuses Offer Hands-on Training Experiences

Students at many sites used similar language to describe their clinical experiences. "We have more bread and butter cases," "we get to do more," "it's very hands-on here," and "we get to do lots of procedures" were common refrains. Students asserted their training was more like the experiences they expected in practice, more "like the real world." Because of heavy patient volumes and strong focus on clinical practice, students were encouraged and expected to actively participate in the wards and ambulatory settings.

This educational environment is a result, in part, of the large patient base at the regional campuses. Administrators often mentioned the "wealth of teaching material." One regional dean noted, "at the main academic medical center, they have 1,200 deliveries each year and 600 students. Here we have 3,600 deliveries and 30 students. You do the math." The medical students at the regional campuses certainly had done these calculations, often mentioning the number of deliveries they had performed on OB/GYN rotations and comparing it to the experiences of fellow students on the main campus.

Faculty and clerkship directors at other campuses also cited the saturation at the main teaching hospital and smaller in-ward patient base. This finding is also consistent with Nutter and Whitcomb's report (2001), which found that

> students may not have an adequate experience in having first contact with patients whom they are able to follow throughout their hospitalization. In some cases, the patient populations that students are exposed to are not optimal for medical students' education. This is more often a problem in major academic medical centers where patients may have very complex, highly specialized problems, and may be critically ill.... Because many patients who formerly would have been cared for in the hospital now receive their care in ambulatory-care settings, the number of patients on inpatient services may be inadequate. (pp. 8-9)

4. Regional Clinical Campuses Allow Creativity and Self-Direction

Students and faculty at the regional campuses stated that, because of size and close teacher-learner interaction, clinical campuses permit creativity and appeal to different learning styles. Some students were attracted to the idea of having a role in planning their educational experience. One third-year student said: "Flexibility is available here. Administrators take the view that 'it's your education.' At the main campus, it's more traditional. The small size here is a benefit. Students are encouraged to plan their own curriculum, to choose electives, and to do something that's never been done before. Creativity is encouraged." Another student appreciated the independent experiences at the regional site: "We get to do things we want to do. We can tailor our education much better. We have independence."

Other students emphasized the differences in pedagogy: "There is a different learning style here. You don't get as many lectures. At the main campus, you learn by reading and by observing. At the regional campus, you learn by doing." Her counterpart said that in choosing where to spend one's clinical years, "It comes down to the way you learn. I have to do it to have it register. Educationally, I'm better off here." A faculty member at another location recognized similarly traits: "Students who come here are more eager, more self-motivated."

Potential downsides exist to this model for certain types of learners. A clerkship director indicated that "students here need to take self-initiative. Sometimes we tell them, 'go find something to do.' Some of them aren't sure what they should do in those cases."

5. Regional Campuses Offer Learner-Focused Culture

Students, faculty, and administrators at the regional campuses emphasized the strong focus on students. The interviewees echoed the theme of cooperation rather than competition. Because of high patient volumes and small numbers of residents, students didn't feel that they had to compete with each other. As a result, said one faculty member, "we get a particular type of student: someone who is looking for something different from the ivory tower. We're a kinder, gentler place, closer to the front lines." This was a theme repeated at other sites. One student who spent time at both campuses stated, "These is a sense of community here; the attendings are more accessible; it's more collegial." Another confirmed, "We are treated nicely here. There are no 'screamers.'" An administrator who worked with both campuses said, "The main campus could learn a lot about how to treat students. The regional faculty are more open and friendly."

Students reacted to this culture in different ways. Most indicated they thrived in such an environment. The potential downside is that an occasional student may be better served in the long run in an environment that challenges his natural tendencies. For example, one student explained that, "Here, you can't get lost. You can't hide. It's easier to be pushed. You don't have to fight you way to the front." While this nurturing environment sounds comfortable, he might in fact benefit more from a competitive environment that broadened his abilities and horizons. Such differences in learning culture underscore the need for administrators and faculty at both campuses to recognize the strengths and weaknesses of different educational settings and to help students choose the one that would serve them best.

6. Regional Campuses Can Offer Unique Educational Foci

At some of the regional campuses, students viewed the organizational structure or focus of the campus as a benefit. For example, several campuses emphasized primary care specialties. For students interested in these areas, the regional campus was an excellent match. Some campuses promoted their community-based focus and close relationships with community physicians in private practice. Again, students who wanted to enter private practice benefited from these relationships by gaining an understanding of that world, perhaps better than they could have by staying in the academic medical center environment. Finally, for a few regional campuses, all the clerkship opportunities were located in one hospital or one small geographic area. In these settings, students reported that they benefited from the continuity by not having to move to a new hospital every six to eight weeks.

Drawbacks

While faculty and students were very positive about the educational experience on the regional campus, they also mentioned downsides.

1. The Educational Experience is not as "Academic"

Many students cited concerns that the regional campus did not have the broad academic resources of the main campus. Students on various campuses reported that the libraries were smaller, fewer electives were offered, fewer opportunities for research were available, and faculty didn't maintain office hours. At some campuses, fewer lectures were offered. One regional dean explained, "We don't have grand rounds in orthopedics or ENT. So our didactic offerings might deter someone interested in subspecialties." On a few campuses, students noted that the lectures were lower quality compared to the main campus. A common complaint at one regional campus was that private physicians sometimes missed their slated lectures. Another disadvantage that students noted was the quality of residents at the branch campus. Many students perceived that the residents did not match their counterparts on the main AHC. "Overall, the residents [at the main site] are more interested in teaching," said one student." Another agreed. "They don't propel you to look at the literature everyday."

These conditions led a few students to believe that some of their colleagues would not enjoy the experience as much as they have. "I think academic-based and scholarly types would hate it here," said one student. Another doubted lab-oriented students would appreciate the clinical campus environment. Most of the branch campuses had little or no research enterprise—although some cited plans to build that infrastructure. (A clear exception was the UMDNJ/RWJ Camden campus, whose FY 2000 total extramural research funding was $82.6 million). Medical students interested in careers as researchers might not find sufficient opportunities at many of the regional sites.

2. Perception of Different Student Outcomes

The second downside cited by students was their concern that the clinical campus experience would be a disadvantage to them in their future careers. Students on one campus said there was a perception that they would be behind in their studies. Many indicated that coming to the regional campus would hurt them in matching for residencies. One said, "I've heard that it impacts getting letters of recommendation. The faculty aren't as well known. There is a prestige factor."

Typically, students heard such concerns before they arrived at the regional campuses. Many students said those concerns were alleviated once they were immersed in the educational program at the branch site. In fact, several fourth-year students indicated that the opportunities at the regional campus helped them in residency interviews by setting them apart from the crowd. One student entering a surgical subspecialty said, "During my surgery clerkship [at the clinical campus], I made my presence known, so I was put in the right place at the right time; I got to operate a lot. I interviewed at 15 places for residency. When asked a surgical question, I was able to answer because I had already done it." Another student said:

[Being at the regional campus is included] in your dean's letter, and you can spin that however you want. I saw it as a huge advantage in setting me apart from all the other applicants that didn't have this type of experience. In the interviews I had, they saw my experience here in a positive way. It was a diverse experience; it gave us something to talk about.

The Role of Technology in the Educational Experience

A brief note can be offered about the role of technology in the delivery and administration of the medical education experience at regional campuses. Many administrators and faculty members indicated that the interaction between the two campuses had improved over the years. One contributing factor has been the availability of new communication technologies. With the advent of email and teleconferencing, students and faculty at multiple locations can communicate much more easily and regularly than in the past. Although the geographic distance is still a real and perceived barrier to integration and communication, that distance is reduced considerably when clerkship directors can exchange ideas via their computer, when students can stay in touch with classmates and faculty members at the main campus, when they can access student services via the internet, and when educational content can be delivered by teleconference. "Videoconferencing has significantly enhanced the frequently and quality of interaction between the two campuses," said one regional department head. A clerkship director maintained, "The acceptance and use of technology has helped improve communication between [the main campus and regional campus]. The distance isn't as big of a deal anymore."

STUDENT RECRUITMENT

Students learn about their options for clinical campuses in various ways. None of the institutions in our study has a highly sophisticated recruitment program as does, say, an undergraduate college and university for high school students. Nor can they, given that their competition would be other campuses of the same medical school. However, the regional campuses do vary in their recruitment efforts.

The most common tact is an informational program on the main campus, in which regional administrators and students provide perspectives about the clinical site. The students in our research focus groups reported these events were sporadically attended and of limited persuasive value (although they are an important first step to get the word out). The programs, events, and activities to which current students responded more positively included:

- *Undergraduate internships, summer programs, or other opportunities* to spend weeks or months immersed at the regional campus before their decision to enroll (and in some cases, before their decision to apply to medical school). For example, UCSF-Fresno runs a Medical Spanish course during the summers. Several students learned about the clinical program during that experience. One student at Alabama had a summer internship in Huntsville and was exposed to the medical school campus.

- *Physical diagnosis courses.* Two clinical campuses (UMDNJ-RWJ Camden and Tufts-Baystate) bring students to campus during their second year for physical diagnosis courses. At Camden, M-3 and M-4 students help teach the course. Current Camden students reported positive outcomes with this arrangement: both to learn from their peers as second-year students and to teach when they were third- and fourth-year students.

- *Field Trips:* Several schools offer "visit" days to attend the regional campus. The success of such programs varied. Several schools reported low attendance for voluntary events. Others require all students to attend.

As noted above, students enrolled at the regional campuses were overwhelmingly satisfied with their experiences. The majority of the ten sites reported strong student interest over the years. But few programs were oversubscribed. Why weren't students beating down the doors to attend the regional campuses?

Many factors come into play, as reported by students and administrators. Logistics affect many students: children enrolled in schools, spouses with jobs, homes already established in the main campus communities. For many medical students, moving to another location after two years is difficult or impossible. For others, guided by inertia, it is simply easier to stay put. As stated earlier, some students who are interested in careers in research or certain subspecialties might prefer the setting of the academic medical center campus.

Others, however, fear the unknown or are guided by misperceptions and myths. An unfortunate situation arises when students for whom the clinical campus program might be a good match do not investigate its offering because of reasons that are not educationally based. Medical schools with clinical campuses should continue to endeavor to provide students with learning opportunities in their first two years to explore options for their clinical training, recognizing different students will choose different learning environments.

FACULTY AT THE REGIONAL CLINICAL CAMPUS

Faculty members at the regional campuses operate at the intersection of academic medicine and private practice. They experience tension in the ambiguous affiliations with their colleagues at the main academic medical center and with private physicians in the regional community.

Certainly these faculty consider themselves academic physicians. They work at the regional campus for the same reasons that faculty members everywhere are drawn to academic medicine:

- "Faculty enjoy the academic setting and environment. That's why they are here. I think many of them would leave if [the medical school] wasn't a player."

- "Part of what we do and who we are is the affiliation with [the medical school]. I don't want to just be a part of a large community practice."

- "I wanted to be at a place where I could teach without the pressure of research for promotion. I didn't want to be in a publish-or-perish environment. I enjoy teaching."

- "I don't want to work for a community hospital. I want to work for a teaching hospital."

- "If there was no affiliation between [the medical school] and [the regional hospital], the hospital would have a hard time recruiting doctors. The academic side is attractive."

In many ways, regional campus faculty are identical to their main campus brethren: drawn to their posts for the ability to teach students and residents;

to work in an academic environment focused on the tripartite mission of teaching, research, and clinical care; and to affiliate with hospitals that embrace these values.

Regional campus faculty, however, expressed less interest in many typical faculty prerogatives. Few regional campuses had faculty senates or governance structures. The vast majority of faculty were not tenured or tenure-eligible. For most, promotion in an academic career ladder was not important: "It's nice on your CV, but it's somewhat meaningless. That's not why we're here." This faculty comment was typical. (Faculty on one campus did express that "there is a culture here for prompting faculty to go through the promotion process and meet the expectations for getting promoted." Such a sentiment, however, was not the norm.)

Regional faculty expressed several reasons for the lack of interest in promotion. First, many are busy clinicians who don't have time to focus on the requirements. Second, they feel little pressure to advance. For example:

- "Responsibilities take too much time. Patient care is still our primary goal. We don't feel pressure to advance; we don't feel a time table."

- "The impetus is personal. There is no pressure from my peers. It is not an expectation in the department."

Third, faculty cited few tangible benefits to promotion. Unlike the case in traditional academic settings, promotion for regional faculty wasn't concomitant with tenure or a salary increase. "They don't make any more money. They do it because of the title change and ego, not for financial remuneration," said one regional dean.

Fourth, many regional campus faculty reported that the promotions process is a time-consuming, cumbersome, and confusing process. Such attitudes are not unique at regional campuses, to be sure, but they are exacerbated by geographic distance and differences in job responsibilities. For example:

- "A major problem is that there's not enough time to get things done. Clinical requirements limit time available for scholarly work. Scholarly activities won't be bench research. Teaching accomplishments count. It's the scholarship of teaching."

- "It's our problem to solve. Because we're a different campus, people here don't realize they're doing creative and scholarly work, even though they are."
- "Before [we had a representative on the main campus' promotion committee], it was a mysterious process for us. It helps to have a representative from the branch campus on that committee."
- "I don't have time to go through the process."
- "Promotion is a cumbersome process. Physicians don't care that much about promotion. They do like to teach, but it's too much of a hassle to apply for appointment and promotion. We need an administrator to take care of that."

Finally, at a few campuses in our study—though not the majority—faculty expressed the perception that they have a more difficult time in the promotion process than do clinical faculty members at the main campus. "Some [main campus] faculty don't fully understand [the regional campus], so it plays into promotion decisions," reported one regional dean. At a campus were clinical faculty are eligible for the tenure track, faculty members reported, "The perception is that it's more difficult for [our] faculty to get tenure and promotion. More folks here convert to a clinical track."

Faculty Development

Another traditional faculty benefit that is less advanced at regional campuses is faculty development programs and opportunities. Few regional campuses have the resources to conduct faculty development programs on their own. They rely on services from the main campus. But the two common factors of time and distance inhibit integration across campuses. First, regional faculty members stated that they didn't have time to participate in faculty development activities because of their demanding clinical schedules. Such concern is not unique to clinical campuses. Second, geographical distance is a barrier. Most regional faculty don't have the inclination to drive several hours for a half-day workshop or one-hour speech. Faculty development offices typically have limited resources and cannot afford to repeat programs on multiple campuses.

Faculty development programs for regional clinical faculty are as vital for the success of the medical education program as for main campus faculty, for the same reasons: opportunities to enhance teaching skills and evaluation techniques, to learn about new educational practices, to expand one's thinking and knowledge. Perhaps, though, faculty development is even more important at a regional campus to develop the faculty's esprit de corps, to build academic culture, and to reward educational excellence in places geographically isolated from the main academic campus. Most of the regional sites in our study were located in communities with other universities. Joint programs between medical school and university neighbors might be one avenue to provide faculty development opportunities to branch campus faculty who otherwise could not participate.

7. The Organizational Relationships Between Main Campus and Branch Campuses

One of our primary purposes for this study was to investigate the organizational and governance relationships between the clinical campus and the main campus. The following section explores these relationships at three levels: at the institutional level, at the departmental level, and the level of curriculum management.

Institutional Relationships

Blended Families

At the highest level, regional clinical campuses are separate, semi-autonomous operating units with responsibility over a wide range of operations and services. Previous literature has described the complex relationships between main campuses and clinical affiliates using the metaphor of marriage (Beljan, 1979; Derzon, 1978). Based on our experience with these ten regional campuses, a different metaphor might be more apt: that of the blended family. Unlike wedded partners, these campuses often didn't chose one another. In many cases, the main campus was a reluctant partner, drawn into the relationship by the pressure of local communities or state politicians. The language used by interviewees speaks to this initial trepidation:

- A regional campus dean: "The president of the university pushed the dean to bring [the regional campus] into the family. The 16 clinical chairs were not ready to embrace that."

- A main campus administrator: "The [clinical campus] faculty felt like little brother with [the main campus] telling them what to do. It took me a long time to get their trust."

Like many blended families, the two entities in many of these medical school relationships—especially the main campus—were cautious, unenthusiastic, or skeptical. The ten campuses in our study varied in how long they have "been together"—from 30 years to three. Some of them reported their interactions with the main campus to be positive and constructive, while others were struggling.

Positive Institutional Dynamics

We identified several factors that appear to influence positive relationships among the main campus and clinical site. First, the clinical site reported they had significant autonomy and didn't feel micromanaged. Second, effective communication channels were opened at many levels. Third, faculty and administrators at the branch campus felt part of the institution because of multiple channels: committee representation; participation in meetings, workshops, forums, and events; consultation by their peers at the main campus; and involvement in decision making. Fourth, the two campuses viewed each other as part of the same whole rather than an "us versus them" mentality. Many of these sentiments were expressed by one branch faculty member who said:

> "There is a mutual respect between the clinical campus and main campus. There is no stepchild feeling at the clinical campus. Competition exists but it's healthy. Faculty members here love teaching; students love the rotations. The campus has autonomy. The main campus doesn't dictate the way everything should be done."

Faculty and administrators spoke positively of their relationship when they perceived the main campus as a peer and equal and when they believed that the main campus viewed them in similar fashion. In other words, the two campus's view of each other depended on mutual admiration. This admiration, in turn, is based—at least in part—on perceptions of prestige. Prestige is "a powerful coin in the academic realm" (Clark, 1987, p. 59). Since the founding of Johns Hopkins University in 1876, Americans have interpreted the model of a "real" university to be focused on research and graduate work (Riesman, 1980). In academic medicine, research-intensive institutions are perceived to be more prestigious than community-based schools; academic clinicians have a higher pecking order than community practitioners. At the regional campuses in our study, those sites with the most positive relationships had congruity with the main campus in hierarchy and prestige: either the branch campus had a substantial research program as did the main site, or both branch and main campus had very small research enterprises. Community-based regional campuses affiliated with very research-intensive main campuses had less constructive relationships because of dissonance in mission, perceptions of prestige, and lack of mutual admiration.

Struggling Relationships

Some regional campuses had a more strained relationship with the main campus. Several factors seemed to contribute to this dynamic.

- The regional campus felt excluded from important decision-making processes. Said one faculty member, "[They] are the horse and we are the cart. When they make changes, they don't necessarily tell us or consult with us. That is complicated because there is no communication."

- The regional campus community perceived a lack of understanding by the main campus. Oftentimes this originated when the regional site was created by legislative fiat without the buy-in from the main campus. "We were grafted onto [the main site] without them having an understanding of what that would mean," said a faculty member. "I think they would unhook us if they could.... There was ambivalence at the beginning." At another campus, the regional dean suggested that "for the most part, [the main campus] doesn't have an appreciation for how this campus works."

Part of this misunderstanding stems from the community-based focus of the regional campuses versus the traditional role of the main academic medical center. At most regional sites, full-time faculty and community physicians are highly interdependent. At traditional academic medical centers, faculty are highly independent of the community. These divergent roles breed mistrust and misunderstanding about roles and values from both ends.

- Faculty at the regional site felt a lack of time to be involved with university affairs. In many cases, the regional faculty had the option to become involved in school-wide committees but their clinical responsibilities prevented it. "So much activity on the branch campus is clinical-oriented," lamented a faculty member, "it's hard for us to cancel a clinic to visit the main site."

- A problem with the "culture of place." Some interviewees asserted that their rural (and therefore less sophisticated and urbane) location of the regional campus affected their perception on the main site. Said a regional dean, "The rank and file faculty [at the main campus] didn't understand our value. They were surprised and disgusted by the affiliation with a poor town [like ours]... They saw the affiliation as being sold down the river."

- The two campuses competed for faculty. At one institution in particular, faculty felt they vied with the main campus over the best talent.

Pragmatism

No institutional relationship was perfect. Those about which interviewees spoke most positively took a pragmatic view of the arrangement. "They are a part of us," said one dean about his regional campus, "and they aren't going away. So we need to make it as good as we can." In many cases, the pragmatic view has developed only after decades of ambivalence. Some main campuses saw the branches—created by state legislators—as draining limited resources. "It's taken 30 years for tensions to fade," said the dean. "Now I view the branch as a fact of life." New faculty and administrators on both campuses brought similar perspectives with them. "The new generation of chairs at the main campus considers us to be part of the package," said a regional dean.

Many regional campuses believe that pragmatic point of view will only grow stronger. With continued changes in healthcare delivery and financing, many of the regional campuses asserted that their importance in medical education will continue to increase. This view is especially true where the main medical school was in a location either removed from significant patient populations or oversaturated with providers. "Their need for us will continue to increase," said one faculty member. "Economic and political factors will make them more like us than us like them," said a colleague on a different campus, hinting at the movement of educational experiences into community-based and outpatient settings. Another faculty member claimed bluntly: "We don't need them but they need us."

Symbolism

The organizational dynamics between main campus and regional campus can be viewed in several ways. There is a structural dimension—for example, how the regional campus is incorporated into the main institution through committees, meetings, and other structures. There is the political dimension—focusing both on power and conflict between the campuses but also on the political benefit each campus offers in dealings with external constituencies. Not to be overlooked, however, is the symbolic aspect of these organizational relationships. Through their actions and interactions, the regional campus and main campus signaled messages about how each viewed the other's importance and role in delivering medical education and clinical care.

Symbolic rituals—the traditional acts and routines that give meaning to human activity—are important in organizations. Bolman and Deal (1991) explained that rituals and ceremonies serve four purposes: "to socialize, to stabilize, to reduce anxieties and ambiguities, and to convey messages to external constituencies" (p. 262). In their everyday dealings with one another, the regional and main campuses at the ten sites used symbols and ritual to fulfill these purposes. For example, at many of the medical schools in our study, the two campuses often would meet half-way between the two cities for annual meetings: Stark, Florida; Stroud, Oklahoma; Flatwoods, West Virginia, to name a few. Surely, these meeting places were not selected for luxury conference centers or other amenities, but rather for the benefit of reduced travel for each group. These meeting places were also highly symbolic. They conveyed to members of the regional campus that they were equal partners with the main site in important decision-making rituals. The annual trek to these remote spots conveyed (literally and figuratively) to the branch campus that "we'll meet you half-way." The absence of such rituals at a few campuses also held symbolic meaning. "It's a one-way street," said one clerkship director, "I'm always going to [the main campus]."

Other small symbolic acts filled important purposes in the organizational relationship. At two campuses, the deans made regular visits to the regional site, weekly or monthly. One dean acknowledged, "It's a symbolic presence. It means a huge deal to the faculty. It says they aren't second class." The other dean maintained an office at the regional campus. Although typically unoccupied, the office conveyed to the regional campus that the dean considered the branch an important part of the school. It suggested that "she wants to know faculty and students." Conversely, the absence of top administrators at some campuses was also noted: "It would be nice for students to see their participation. It would send the message that [we] were important."

The symbolism of decision making impacted many regional sites. Many pointed to educational innovations that germinated at the branch campus and then blossomed at the main campus. These curricular improvements were important for the positive impact on medical students, to be sure. But they also were important because they signaled to the faculty at the regional campus that their contributions were significant and valuable. Phoenix-based members of the curriculum committee at the University of Arizona, for example, convinced the committee that all students should be required to have ophthalmoscopes. According to interviewees at the branch campus, this decision had two important symbolic components for Phoenix faculty. First, it signaled that Tucson faculty listened to them and valued their suggestions. Second, it demonstrated that the Phoenix faculty were committed to medical education.

Finally, the symbolism of titles and their uses affected organizational dynamics. At Oklahoma, the title of the chief executive of the Tulsa campus is "dean," not associate or assistant dean. For the Tulsa campus community, this title indicated the equality of the two campuses as well as the autonomy in local decision making. At another campus, regional faculty have faculty titles but aren't allowed to use university letterhead. For them, the regulations suggested that they weren't full-fledged members of the campus community.

These examples suggest that the symbolism of everyday events can hold enormous import in system-wide cohesiveness and organizational effectiveness. In each of these medical schools, the relationship between main campus and branch campus was not only predicated on institutional resources and politics. Additionally, the dynamic was based on rituals, ceremony, and perception that filled the void of organizational uncertainty and ambiguity. Small symbolic acts sent important messages to the regional campus about institutional identity—about "who we are."

The Paradox of Distance

The separation of many miles created an interesting paradox for the regional sites in their interactions with the main campus. On one hand, the regional campus communities craved autonomy; on the other, they wanted attention. The geographic distance between the two campuses both fostered and inhibited their needs.

At the institutional level, many interviewees spoke about their desire to be left alone. Examples of this sentiment were pervasive:

- "We like autonomy. The main campus doesn't impose much on us."

- "We don't want too much attention."
- "I like the fact that they leave us alone."
- "There is a sense of autonomy here. We like it that way."

The considerable mileage between campuses facilitated this independence. Senior administrators at the main sites were only present on occasion, leaving the regional campus to govern its own affairs.

On the other hand, the members of the regional campuses didn't like the fact that the physical distance created barriers to understanding, appreciation, and participation on the main campus. For example, a regional faculty member received one of 100 university-wide awards for excellence in teaching; the award was a laptop computer. But in order to receive the laptop, he was required to go to the main university campus for training. A busy clinician, he didn't have the time to travel the distance to attend training, so he never received the computer. The main campus attitude of not making accommodations for their needs and circumstances "is sometimes frustrating," he said. Another regional faculty member noted that his main campus department chair makes an annual appearance and "mispronounces our names." An associate dean cited the lack of attention by the main campus: "The associate chairs [at the regional campus] and the chairs [at the main campus] wouldn't know it if they ran into each other in the airport."

Geographical separation created a paradox of "love me and leave me alone" at many of the regional campuses. Many regional clinical campuses wanted both independence and attention. Interviewees cited benefits and weaknesses to the geographical distance between the two sites. "If you ask what's good and bad about the relationship?" one regional dean posed. "Seventy miles. That's the answer to both." A department chair at another institution said similarly: "Do we want more or less interaction? Yes."

Balanced Leadership

A final theme that emerged from our analysis of organizational relationships at the institutional level was the primacy of balanced leadership between the chief executives at the regional and main campus. For some schools, the regional community viewed the main site as exercising "bungee" leadership: "They come in, they create an uproar, then they disappear. After things settle down, the process repeats. This undermines the governance of the local dean." Regional campuses and their parent campuses had to negotiate a balance between local autonomy and school-wide control. At some sites, the structure of the organization didn't effectively facilitate that balance. For example, one regional dean had the financial responsibility for the entire clinical campus, but none of the local department chairs reported to him for their clinical services. Schools that achieved this balance had equilibrium between local decision making and central authority. One main campus dean asserted, "The dean of the regional campus has to have autonomy while still reporting to the dean. In a crisis, the main dean is in charge. But the regional dean has to have power in and of himself. That requires trust."

Departmental Relationships

Relationships between departments on the regional clinical campus and the main campus were highly variable. Even within the same school, some regional chairs reported close-knit interactions and others cited no relationship at all. The chairs most often attributed this variation to two factors: (1) personal relationships between the department heads and (2) shared teaching or research.

In many cases when the departmental relationship was considered positive or strong, the two department heads had previous professional or personal relationships. On several occasions, regional faculty members had once worked at the main site and knew their colleagues well. One main campus department chair had been the chair at the regional campus. In other cases, the departments collaborated on mission-related activities. One regional department head was co-chair of a Gamma knife program at the main site. He reported very close interaction. Some chairs noted strong relationships because of jointly developed teaching projects. Said one, "We are all very actively involved with each other in research and teaching."

Several themes emerged as enablers of productive cross-departmental links. First, the regional department perceived a sense of equality and respect among members in both locations. Similar to productive relationships at the institutional level, there was a willingness for departments to meet halfway between both campuses or to alternate meeting locations on each site. Second, active and regular communication took place. Some departments had department-wide meetings for all faculty several times a year.

Others held monthly or bimonthly meetings by teleconference. Third, the regional departments felt they positively contributed to the mission of the department and felt their contributions were valued. "We've developed innovations they have not," said one chair. "[The department at the main campus] sees tremendous value in our participation," said another. Fourth, chairs at both sites were expected by the dean and regional dean to engage in collaboration for medical education and scholarship.

More often, however, chairs at the regional campus reported little or no interaction. Echoing the attitudes of the majority of regional chairs in the study, one noted: "We don't have any regular contact with the [main campus] department. We try to have a collegial relationship but don't have any regular contact."

There were several impediments to inter-campus interaction at the departmental level. First, cultural differences—perceived or real—existed. The regional chairs often saw wide gaps between their clinical orientation and the research focus of the main site. One regional chair claimed, "We're really not on their map because [the main campus department] is subspecialty-oriented. Their view is that students who want to be subspecialists need to spend their third and fourth year around research." Other cultural differences were noted between the traditional tertiary academic medical center at the main campus and the community-based approach at the regional campus. A chair said, "They worry we are contaminating students with lowbrow community experiences." A second impediment was distance. Despite advances in telecommunications, the distance between the two locations inhibited better interaction. Third, the clinical faculty at the regional campus sometimes felt too busy to participate in departmental meetings, committees, or other events.

At the majority of schools in our study, the regional department head was an "associate chair" who reported to the chair at the main site. Two schools, however, had different arrangements. University of Oklahoma and Mercer University maintain separate chairs at each site—there is no reporting relationship between the two. Mercer explains this organizational relationship as follows:

> The July 1, 1999 Agreement with Memorial Health University Medical Center provides for academic clinical departments at both the Savannah campus and the Macon campus.... The primary

advantage of separate clinical departments is that the organization and operation of the Savannah campus is now more easily handled between the Savannah-based administration, department chairs, and Savannah-based faculty, rather than through department chairs in Macon. The 150-mile geographic distance between the two clinical campuses limited the day-to-day interaction between the Macon department chairs and Savannah-based faculty. The development of separate departments was a practical solution to the communication and operational issues created by the geographic distance between Macon and Savannah.... Chairs report to the Associate Dean for Savannah Programs for day-to-day operational and academic issues. Chairs have overall responsibility and reporting relationship to the dean of the School of Medicine.

The level of interest and interaction also can be based on another structural element: financial arrangements. At the University of Alabama, for example, funds flow directly to the regional campus in Huntsville; no funding for the branch comes through the department chairs in Birmingham. A Huntsville administrator noted, "Their interest is commensurate with funding." The Tulsa chairs also noted this financial separation: "We have a separate budget. There is no reporting relationship, so we are a real campus with real chairs."

Curriculum Management

The most satisfaction, congruity, and synergy in the relationships between the main and regional campuses came at the level of education and curriculum management, as expressed by clerkship directors and assistant deans for education at the regional sites. These close-knit relationships at this level are not surprising, perhaps, given the accreditation requirements of the LCME. Clerkship directors across sites—near and geographically separate—must ensure the comparability of the educational experience, which necessitates that they work together. But several additional factors—beyond mandated regulations—contributed to the positive experiences among participants at this level.

First, members of the regional campus were actively engaged in the school-wide curriculum committees. They participated in meetings and decision-making often through in-person meetings, email communication, and teleconferencing. Although many interviewees noted that electronic communications are not equal substitutes for in-person participation, they felt those technologies allowed them to participate in the medical education program at the school. Second, regional clerkship directors felt their contributions were valued and appreciated. They felt on par with their colleagues at the main site. One regional clerkship director observed, "They want our input. They value us as we do them. We're just as vital as they are."

Two campuses reported less satisfaction with curriculum issues than the others. In both cases, the interviewees noted wide variation in clerkship interaction—similar to the variation at the department level. "There is no standard expectation in the dean's office." One clerkship director reported, "We don't have regular meetings with [their counterparts at the main campus.] We have a high degree of autonomy." A director of undergraduate medical education at a regional campus didn't find the same spirit of camaraderie that other campuses reported: "I'm always going there. There's not much of a 'let me help you' attitude."

Summary of the Organizational Relationships between Main and Regional Campuses: The "Bridge" Culture

During the wrap-up to one of our visits, a regional dean posed the question: "Are we an island or a peninsula?" The question spoke to the complex relationships that these regional campuses maintain with the main medical school campus. On one hand they are seemingly independent and autonomous. Many branch campuses fly beneath the main campus' radar. "Out of sight, out of mind" might be an appropriate adage. On the other hand, these regional campuses are definitively a sub-unit of the whole. They are not independently accredited; they cannot directly admit students; they do not award degrees. These sites are quite different from, say, a multi-campus state system like the University of California, in which the separate campuses truly are "islands."

The answer to the "island or peninsula" question, therefore, is neither. They are neither fully part of the main academic medical center nor truly separate, not fully independent nor fully integrated. Regional faculty are not fully incorporated into the ranks of academic physicians but neither are they private clinicians.

Instead, the regional campus is a bridge. These campuses link the academic setting to the community, research to practice, one region of the state to another. They display cultures of being "in-between"—as expressed in the paradox of wanting to be recognized as part of the medical school yet autonomous at the same time. They are not fully part of either community—the distant academic or the local. "The main campus doesn't have an appreciation for us" was a common refrain. But so too was a lack of understanding by the local community. One regional dean relayed the following story: "I was wearing a shirt with the logo of the faculty physician group at a local hotel. A resident commented, 'Oh, I didn't know there was a university campus here in town.' I asked if she was new to the area. 'No,' she said, 'I've lived here all my life.'"

These campuses are neither islands nor peninsulas: they are isthmuses, connecting different cultures, different values, and different regions. They share a "bridge" culture at the nexus of education and patient care, of academic and clinician, of ivory tower and community. They are to be valued for expanding opportunities, experiences, and missions, and for bridging the oftentimes wide gulf between town and gown.

8. Conclusions

We endeavored to provide an understanding of the purposes, scope of operations, organizational arrangements, and management issues of geographically separate clinical campuses affiliated with U.S. medical schools. There are two findings in particular we wish to reiterate here.

The first observation is that students who attend the regional campuses for their clinical education are a satisfied lot. They believe that the educational experiences provided at regional clinical campus sites are as good as, if not better than, the educational experiences provided in major teaching hospitals. They believe that they encounter a wider range of clinical conditions, have the opportunity to perform more clinical procedures, and receive more individual clinical instruction from both residents and faculty members than would be the case if they were assigned to their medical school's major teaching hospital.

Second, even though the ten regional sites in our study varied considerably in their organization, scope of operations, and administrative relationships between regional campus and the main medical school campus, this organizational variation did not appear to affect students' positive perceptions. The praise for the educational experience was universal, whether the campus was large or small, isolated or integrated, urban or rural. The constant across these ten regional campuses was that the sites were patient-centered and student-focused.

While little published literature has focused on these entities in the past, regional clinical campuses play an important role in medical education in the United States. Thomas Jefferson, writing to Joseph Cabell in May 1824, offered what is perhaps the earliest known rationale for a regional clinical campus for a medical school:

> No, Sir; Richmond is no place to furnish subjects for clinical lectures. I have always had Norfolk in view for this purpose. The climate and pontine country around Norfolk render it truly sickly in itself. It is, moreover, the rendezvous not only of the shipping of commerce, but of the vessels of the public navy. The United States have there a hospital already established, and supplied with subjects from these local circumstances. I had thought and have mentioned to yourself and

our colleagues, that when our medical school has got well under way, we should propose to the federal government the association with that establishment, and at our own expense, of the clinical branch of our medical school, so that our students, after qualifying themselves with the other branches of the science here, might complete their course of preparation by attending clinical lectures for six or twelve months at Norfolk.

In what is amazingly prescient, Jefferson highlights the benefits of a clinical branch: the ability to expand clinical training opportunities using existing hospitals; the integration of interested organizations to build partnerships for mutual benefit; and an adequate patient base for the effective delivery of a clinical curriculum. The circumstances haven't changed much in 200 years. Medical schools that have regional campuses must continue to value their contributions, understand their unique circumstances, and integrate them into the family of academic medicine. More clinical campuses are on the horizon. Medical school leaders can learn lessons from the existing sites to create effective organizational relationships among main and branch campuses, so that medical students who attend both campuses receive nothing less than excellence in their clinical education.

Appendix 1

Basic Science Branch Campuses at U.S. Medical Schools

Indiana University School of Medicine
Bloomington
Evansville
Fort Wayne
West Lafayette
Muncie
Gary
South Bend
Terre Haute

UCLA, David Geffin School of Medicine
UC-Riverside

University of California, San Francisco
UC-Berkeley

University of Illinois at Chicago College of Medicine
Urbana-Champaign (also considered a clinical branch campus)

University of Minnesota Medical School
Duluth (as of 2004, Duluth will no longer be separately accredited)

University of Washington School of Medicine
Anchorage, AL
Moscow, ID
Bozeman, MT
Pullman, WA
Laramie, WY

Appendix 2
Geographically Separate Campuses (Basic and Clinical Campuses) Included in Various Classification Schemes

	Main Campus	Geographically Separate Location	LCME*	Watt, et al. (1993)	Swick (2000)	DAME (2002)
1	Case Western Reserve	Detroit	No	No	Yes	Yes
2	Dartmouth Medical School	Providence	No	Yes	No	Yes
3	East Tennessee State University	Kingsport	Yes	No		Yes
		Bristol	Yes	No		Yes
		Rogersville	Yes	No	Yes	Yes
		Mountain City	Yes	No		Yes
		Chattanooga	No	No		Yes
4	Indiana University	Bloomington	No	Yes		Yes
		Evansville	No	Yes		Yes
		Fort Wayne	No	Yes		Yes
		Gary	No	Yes		Yes
		West Lafayette	No	Yes	Yes	Yes
		Muncie	No	Yes		Yes
		South Bend	No	Yes		Yes
		Terre Haute	No	Yes		Yes
5	LSU--New Orleans	Baton Rouge	No	No	Yes	Yes
6	Mayo Medical School	Scottsdale, AZ	Yes	Yes	Yes	Yes
		Jacksonville, FL	Yes	Yes		Yes
7	MCP Hahnemann (Drexel)	Allegheny	No	Yes	No	Yes
		Monmouth Medical Center (NJ)	No	No		Yes
8	Mercer University School of Medicine	Savannah	Yes	No	Yes	Yes
9	Michigan State University	Flint	Yes	Yes		Yes
		Grand Rapids	Yes	Yes		Yes
		Kalamazoo	Yes	Yes	Yes	Yes
		Saginaw	Yes	Yes		Yes
		Upper Peninsula (Marquette)	Yes	Yes		Yes
10	New York Medical College	Westchester County	No	Yes	No	Yes
11	Northeastern Ohio University	Akron	Yes	Yes		Yes
		Canton	Yes	Yes	Yes	Yes
		Youngstown	Yes	Yes		Yes
		Barberton	Yes	No		Yes
12	Penn State Medical College	Lehigh Valley	No	No	No	Yes
		York	No	No		Yes
13	Southern Illinois University	Carbondale	No	Yes	No	Yes
14	SUNY Upstate Medical University	Binghamton	Yes	Yes	Yes	Yes
15	Temple	West Penn Hospital, Pittsburgh	Yes	No	No	Yes
16	Texas A&M University	Temple	No	Yes	Yes	Yes
17	Texas Tech University	Amarillo	Yes	Yes	Yes	Yes
		El Paso	Yes	Yes		Yes
		Odessa	Yes	No		Yes
18	Tufts	Baystate Medical Center, Springfield MA	No	No	No	Yes

	Main Campus	Geographically Separate Location	LCME*	Watt, et al. (1993)	Swick (2000)	DAME (2002)
19	UCLA	Drew	Yes	No	Yes	Yes
		Riverside	Yes	No	Yes	Yes
20	UCSF	Fresno	Yes	Yes	Yes	Yes
		Berkeley	Yes	No	Yes	No
21	UMDNJ/Robert Wood Johnson Medical School	Camden	Yes	Yes	Yes	Yes
22	University of Alabama	Huntsville	Yes	Yes	Yes	Yes
		Tuscaloosa	Yes	Yes		Yes
23	University of Arizona	Phoenix, AZ	Yes	Yes	Yes	Yes
24	University of Arkansas	Fayetteville	No	No	Yes	Yes
25	University of Florida	Talahassee	No	Yes	Yes	Yes
		Jacksonville	Yes	Yes	Yes	Yes
26	University of Illinois	Peoria	Yes	Yes	Yes	Yes
		Rockford	Yes	Yes		Yes
		Urbana-Champaign	Yes	Yes		Yes
27	University of Iowa	Des Moines	No	No	Yes	Yes
28	University of Kansas	Wichita	Yes	Yes	Yes	Yes
29	University of Louisville	Madisonville	No	No	Yes	Yes
30	University of Minnesota, Duluth	Minneapolis	No	Yes	Yes	Yes
31	University of Nevada	Las Vegas	Yes	Yes	No	Yes
32	University of North Dakota	Bismark	Yes	Yes	Yes	Yes
		Fargo	Yes	Yes		Yes
		Minot	No	Yes		Yes
33	University of Oklahoma	Tulsa	Yes	Yes	Yes	Yes
34	University of South Carolina	Greenville	Yes	No	No	Yes
35	University of South Dakota	Yankton	Yes	Yes	Yes	Yes
		Rapid City/West River	Yes	Yes		Yes
		Vermillion	Yes	Yes		Yes
36	University of Tennessee, Memphis	Jackson	No	Yes	Yes	Yes
		Knoxville	Yes	No		Yes
		Chattanooga	Yes	No		Yes
37	University of Texas Medical Branch	Austin	No	No	No	Yes
38	University of Vermont	Portland, ME	Yes	No	Yes	Yes
39	University of Virginia	Roanoke	Yes	No	No	Yes
40	University of Washington (WWAMI)	Moscow, ID	Yes	Yes	Yes	Yes
		Pullman, WA	Yes	Yes		Yes
		Bozeman, MT	Yes	Yes		Yes
		Fairbanks/Anchorage, AK	Yes	Yes		Yes
		Laramie, WY	No	No		Yes
41	University of Wisconsin	Milwaukee	No	No	Yes	Yes
		Western Clinical Campus	No	No		Yes
42	West Virginia University	Charleston	Yes	Yes	No	Yes

* = refers to schools that designate a "geographically separated campus" on their LCME Database, section II/III, F, 23-25.

Appendix 3

Survey of Regional Clinical Campuses Sent to Associate Deans of Medical Education

1. What is the title of the senior official at the clinical campus responsible for medical education programs?_____

2. To whom on the main campus does this person report?_____

3. In what year was this clinical campus started?_____

4. Do document(s) exist that explain the purpose for the establishment of this clinical campus?
   - ❏ Yes, document(s) exist
   - ❏ No, documents do not exist
   - ❏ Don't know

5. Which required third-year clerkships are offered at this clinical campus? Check all that apply:
   - ❏ Internal medicine
   - ❏ Obstetrics & gynecology
   - ❏ Pediatrics
   - ❏ Psychiatry
   - ❏ Surgery
   - ❏ Family medicine

6. We are interested in learning how students are assigned or elect to attend the clinical campus. Which of the following describes the arrangements at your institution?

   - ❏ Third-year medical students who attend the clinical campus do so for the full-year. No students rotate in or out for specific clerkships.
     What percentage of the 3rd-year class attends for the full year? _____%

   - ❏ Some third-year medical students attend the clinical campus for the full year and other students rotate in and out for specific clerkships.
     What percentage of the 3rd-year class attends for the full year? _____%

   - ❏ No third-year medical students attend the clinical campus for the full year, but students rotate in and out for specific clerkships.

   - ❏ Other. Please describe._____

7. Does the medical school provide any funds to the clinical campus for the education of medical students at the clinical site?

   - ❏ Yes. If so, how much funding is transferred? _____
   - ❏ No

Appendix 4

Regional Clinical Campuses Affiliated with Traditional Medical Schools (i.e. Non-Community Based)

Medical School	Clinical Campus
1. Drexel	1. Allegheny General Hospital, Pittsburgh
	2. Monmouth Medical Center, Long Branch, NJ
2. Mercer	3. Memorial Health University Medical Center, Savannah
3. Penn State	4. Lehigh Valley Medical Center, Allentown
	5. York Hospital, York
4. SUNY Upstate	6. Binghamton
5. Temple	7. West Penn Hospital, Pittsburgh
6. Tufts	8. Baystate Medical Center, Springfield
7. UMDNJ – Robert Wood Johnson	9. Camden
8. University of Alabama	10. Huntsville
	11. Tuscaloosa
9. University of Arizona	12. Phoenix
10. UC-San Francisco	13. Fresno
11. University of Florida	14. Jacksonville
12. University of Illinois – Chicago	15. Peoria
	16. Rockford
	17. Urbana-Champaign (basic & clinical)
13. University of Iowa	18. Des Moines
14. University of Kansas	19. Wichita
15. University of Oklahoma	20. Tulsa
16. University of Tennessee	21. Chattanooga
	22. Knoxville
17. University of Texas MB	23. Austin
18. University of Virginia	24. Roanoke
19. University of Wisconsin	25. Western Clinical Campus (Lacrosse)
20. West Virginia University	26. Charleston

Appendix 5

Regional Campuses Included in Site Visits

- Mercer University School of Medicine—Savannah campus (Memorial Health University Hospital)

- SUNY Upstate Medical University—Binghamton campus

- Tufts University School of Medicine—Baystate Medical Center campus (Springfield, MA)

- UMDNJ Robert Wood Johnson Medical School—Camden campus (Cooper Hospital/University Medical Center)

- University of Alabama School of Medicine—Huntsville campus

- University of Arizona College of Medicine—Phoenix campus

- University of California, San Francisco School of Medicine—Fresno campus

- University of Florida College of Medicine—Jacksonville campus

- University of Oklahoma College of Medicine—Tulsa campus

- West Virginia University School of Medicine—Charleston campus

Appendix 6

Site Visit Schedule

Site Visit Information
A two-member team from the AAMC is conducting site visits at ten regional medical school campuses in Spring 2002. The purpose of these visits is to understand the structure, organization, operations, and management of clinical campuses of U.S. medical schools.

During our site visit, we would like to interview the following individuals and/or groups:
- Regional dean
- Hospital director
- Elected president of the organized medical staff
- Other key administrators
- Focus group with students (preferably with each of the clerkships represented)
- Focus group with several members of the core faculty

We would ask that a designated contact person at your site help arrange the interview times and places with each of the individual/groups.

Proposed Interview Schedule
The following proposed schedule will hopefully provide a framework for each site, with the understanding that it will be altered to accommodate individual schedules, unique institutional characteristics, and your preferences. Please let us know if there are additional people you'd like to include in the site visit schedule.

8 – 9:30am	Meeting with regional dean and anyone else he/she would like to invite. Purpose: to provide an overview of regional campus and its programs and operations.
9:30 – 10am	Hospital CEO or other executive
10 - 10:30am	President of organized medical staff or other medical staff representative

10:30 – 11am and 11 – 11:30am	One-half hour interviews with two different clerkship directors
11:30 – 11:45am	Break/Buffer time to remain on schedule
11:45 – 1:15pm	Lunch meeting with students
1:15 – 2pm	Faculty focus group
2 – 2:30pm	Wrap up with regional dean

Written information

Prior to our visit, we would like to obtain written information that will help us understand the current and historical context of the clinical campus. While the specific types of written material will vary by campus, we are interested in items such as:

- Faculty policies/handbook specific to the regional campus
- Student "marketing" materials (i.e., information distributed to medical students explaining the facilities, services, and operations of the regional campus)
- Student policies/handbook specific to the regional campus
- Strategic planning documents
- Documents/materials about why the regional campus started
- Financial statement
- Relevant portions of LCME self-study reports
- Other relevant information

Appendix 7

Interview Guide

Regional Dean:
1. What is the history of regional campus? Do any historical developments affect how the campus is organized today?
2. What is your background?
3. Describe your interaction with the dean. How often do you go to the main campus? How often does the dean visit the regional campus?
4. What is your impression of how this regional campus is perceived by important decision-makers on the main campus?
5. To what degree are administrators at the main campus informed and knowledgeable about the management and operations of this regional campus?
6. What are the sources of your salary support?
7. How are the medical student programs funded?
8. How are students recruited?
9. What other people on the main campus do you interact with?
10. How many full-time faculty are at the regional campus? How are they appointed? Promoted?
11. Are there part-time faculty appointments?
12. Are there conflicts between private physicians and faculty?
13. How are regional faculty integrated into the medical school faculty? What differences do they face?

Hospital administrators:
1. Why have a formal relationship with the medical school? What's the motivating force?
2. For CEO: How do you view the affiliation?
3. How does the affiliation fit into the strategic vision of the hospital?
4. Where would you like the relationship to be in 5-10 years?
5. How do community physicians view this affiliation?
6. In what ways, if any, does the hospital integrate the affiliation into its marketing?
7. What are the benefits of the relationship for the hospital? Does the medical student program add anything?
8. How does medical education affect the hospital's revenue and expenditures?

Elected president of medical staff:
1. How do you view the affiliation?
2. What is your level of involvement?
3. How do community physicians view the affiliation?

4. Are there town-gown problems?
5. Is there competition between university physicians and community physicians?
6. What do the medical students do for the hospital?
7. How does the surrounding community view the affiliation?

Clerkship coordinators:
1. What type of interchange is there at the department level between main and regional campus?
2. What contrast exist between the two sites?
3. What does the regional site do for the main campus? Could the main campus department do without the program at the regional site?
4. How much freedom and flexibility do you have in decisions?
5. What's the biggest challenge?
6. What brings faculty to the campus?

Department chiefs:
1. How would you characterize the relationship between this campus and the main campus of the medical school?
2. How would you characterize the relationship with the hospital?
3. What does the regional site do for the main campus?

Faculty:
1. What is your experience with the appointment and promotion process? Do you perceive differences in this process at the regional campus and main campus? Is there a regional campus representative on the main campus APT committee?
2. What concerns, if any, do regional faculty have with the promotions process?
3. Are there faculty development services at the regional campus?
4. Is there an academic senate at the regional site? Representation on the academic senate at the main site?
5. How do you think faculty at the main campus perceive faculty from this campus?

Students:
1. How did you hear about the regional campus program?
2. What did you hear about it?
3. Why did you come?
4. What has been your experience?
5. What are the positives and negatives of attending a regional clinical campus?
6. What would you recommend to others?
7. How would you characterize interaction with attending physicians? With residents?
8. If you could make changes to the program, would you? If so, what?

Appendix 8

**Survey Sent to Known Population of Regional Clinical Campuses
(Including those affiliated with community-based medical schools
and traditional medical schools)**

Survey of Regional Clinical Campuses

Thank you for taking time to respond to this brief questionnaire. As part of its study on regional clinical campuses at U.S. medical schools, the AAMC is compiling data on the organization and scope of operations of these regional campuses. Your participation is vital to understand the range of characteristics of the many regional campuses in the country. The information collected herein will be considered unrestricted, which means it may be published with individual school identification.

Please use whichever method is most convenient to return the survey by **June 14, 2002**:

ELECTRONIC   Complete the electronic copy of the survey and email it as an attachment to wmallon@aamc.org

PAPER/FAX   Complete the paper copy of the survey and FAX it to 202-828-1125, attention: William T. Mallon

PAPER/MAIL   Complete the paper copy of the survey and MAIL it to: William T. Mallon, AAMC, 2450 N Street, NW, Washington DC 20037

General Information

1. Name of regional campus:

2. In what year did the regional campus start?

3. Title of the senior medical school official (i.e., regional dean) at this campus:

4. Name of person currently holding this position:

5. To whom at the main campus does this person report (name and title)?

6. For the regional dean's salary, please indicate the approximate percentage of support from each source:

    Medical school/university: _____%
    Hospital: _____%
    Faculty practice plan: _____%
    Other (please specify):   _____%
    = 100%

7. *Excluding* the regional dean, how many administrative personnel (FTE) are employed *by the medical school* at the regional campus? (Please include the FTE for faculty with part-time assignments [e.g. assistant deans] as well as full-time administrative personnel.)
   _____

8. Does the regional campus have an organizational chart detailing its administrative structure?
   ❏ Yes   ❏ No

9. Do other health-related schools/colleges of the university offer programs at this campus?
   ❏ Yes   ❏ No

   9a. If yes, please check all that apply:
   ❏ Nursing   ❏ Pharmacy   ❏ Dentistry   ❏ Allied Health
   ❏ Public Health   ❏ Physician Assistant   ❏ Other:_____

10. Please indicate the approximate amount of external research funding received annually from all sources at this regional medical school campus.
    - Less than $2.5 million
    - $2.5-$5 million
    - $5-$10 million
    - Over $10 million

11. How many faculty members at the regional site have NIH grants?_____

12. Do faculty member at the regional campus have representation on the following committees at the main medical school campus:

Committee	Representation?	If yes, are faculty reps elected or appointed?
Tenure/Promotion	❏ Yes ❏ No	❏ Elected ❏ Appointed
Curriculum	❏ Yes ❏ No	❏ Elected ❏ Appointed
Admissions	❏ Yes ❏ No	❏ Elected ❏ Appointed
Student progress/review	❏ Yes ❏ No	❏ Elected ❏ Appointed

13. Does the regional campus have its own promotion and tenure committee, separate from the main campus?
    ❏ Yes   ❏ No

Student Arrangements

14. Which required third-year clerkships are offered at this clinical campus? Check all that apply.
    - ❑ Internal medicine
    - ❑ Surgery
    - ❑ Psychiatry
    - ❑ Pediatrics
    - ❑ Obstetrics & gynecology
    - ❑ Family medicine

15. Which of the following describes the arrangements for third-year students at the regional clinical campus?
    - ❑ Third-year medical students who attend the clinical campus do so for the full-year. No students rotate in or out for required clerkships.
      What percentage of the entire 3rd-year medical school class attends this regional clinical campus for the full year?_____%

    - ❑ Some third-year medical students attend the clinical campus for the full year and other students rotate in and out for required clerkships.
      What percentage of the entire 3rd-year medical school class attends this regional clinical campus for the full year?_____%

    - ❑ No third-year medical students attend the clinical campus for the full year, but students rotate in and out for required clerkships. (**Please skip to question 18**)

    - ❑ Other. Please describe._____

Complete questions 16 & 17 only if a portion of 3rd-year students attend for the full year

16. If third-year student attend the clinical campus for the full year, how are they assigned to this campus? (e.g. voluntary choice, assignment, lottery system, etc.)
    _____
    _____
    _____

17. At what point in time do students learn of their assignment to this clinical campus?
    - ❑ At the time of admission into the medical school
    - ❑ In their first year
    - ❑ In their second year

Affiliated Hospitals and Residencies

18. Please list the hospital(s) affiliated with the regional clinical campus at which third-year students complete clerkship rotations. (Please do not include ambulatory sites.)

19. Are residency programs offered by the affiliated hospitals at this regional clinical campus?
    ❏ Yes   ❏ No **(Please skip to question 22)**

20. Please list the accredited residency programs that are offered at the hospital(s) affiliated with this regional clinical campus.

21. The residency programs at this clinical campus are sponsored by:
    ❏ The medical school, with the same ACGME institutional sponsor number at the main medical school campus

    ❏ The medical school, with a different ACGME institutional sponsor number from the main medical school campus

    ❏ The hospital(s) affiliated with the regional clinical campus.

Faculty

23. Please indicate the number of individuals with faculty appointments at the regional campus:
    Full-time:
    Part-time:
    Volunteer:

Questions 23-26 regard full-time faculty:

23. What are the employment arrangements for the majority of full-time clinical faculty members at the regional campus who are active in medical practice?
    ❏ These faculty are employed solely by the medical school/university

    ❏ These faculty members are employed solely by a practice group or hospital(s)/health system affiliated with the regional clinical campus

    ❏ These faculty members are employed both by the medical school/university and a separate practice group or hospital/health system

24. The majority of full-time clinical faculty members are compensated through the issuance of:
    ❏ One paycheck, which compensates for activities in all missions

    ❏ Two or more paychecks, one from the medical school/university and one or more from a practice group or hospital/health system

25. How many full-time clinical faculty are appointed to the following tracks?

Type of appointment	Number of full-time faculty
Tenured	
Tenure-track/tenure-eligible	
Non-tenure-track/clinical track	
Other (specify)	

26. Is there a faculty practice plan for full-time faculty at the regional campus?
    ❏ Yes   ❏ No

    26a. If yes, is the faculty practice plan at the regional campus separate from the faculty practice plan at the main medical school campus?
    ❏ Yes, the faculty practice plan at the regional site is separate from the main medical school campus.

    ❏ No, faculty members at the regional site are members of the faculty practice plan at the main medical school site.

SURVEY RESPONDENT INFORMATION

27. Please provide the following information for the person who completed this survey:
    Name
    Title
    Phone
    Email

Appendix 9

Known Population of U.S. Regional Clinical Campuses
(including those affiliated with traditional and community-based medical schools)

Medical School	Clinical Campus
1. Drexel	1. Allegheny General Hospital, Pittsburgh
	2. Monmouth Medical Center, Long Branch, NJ
2. Mercer	3. Memorial Health University Medical Center, Savannah
3. Penn State	4. Lehigh Valley Medical Center, Allentown
	5. York Hospital, York
4. SUNY Upstate	6. Binghamton
5. Temple	7. West Penn Hospital, Pittsburgh
6. Tufts	8. Baystate Medical Center, Springfield
7. UMDNJ – RWJ	9. Camden
8. University of Alabama	10. Huntsville
	11. Tuscaloosa
9. University of Arizona	12. Phoenix
10. UC-San Francisco	13. Fresno
11. University of Florida	14. Jacksonville
12. University of Illinois – Chicago	15. Peoria
	16. Rockford
	17. Urbana-Champaign (basic & clincial)
13. University of Iowa	18. Des Moines
14. University of Kansas	19. Wichita
15. University of Oklahoma	20. Tulsa
16. University of Tennessee	21. Chattanooga
	22. Knoxville
17. University of Texas MB	23. Austin
18. University of Virginia	24. Roanoke
19. University of Wisconsin	25. Western Clinical Campus (LaCrosse)
	26. Milwaukee
20. West Virginia University	27. Charleston

21. Michigan State University   28. Flint
29. Grand Rapids
30. Kalamazoo
31. Saginaw
32. Upper Peninsula Program (Marquette)

22. Texas Tech University   33. Amarillo
34. El Paso
35. Odessa

23. University of North Dakota   36. Fargo
37. Southwest Campus (Bismarck)
38. Northwest Campus (Minot)

24. University of South Carolina   39. Greenville
25. University of South Dakota   40. Yankton
41. West River (Rapid City)

Others Not in Official Count

Not Operational at Time of Study

University of Texas – San Antonio	Harlingen *(opened July 2002)*
Virginia Commonwealth University	Fairfax *(under development)*
West Virginia University	Martinsburg *(under development)*

Determined Not to Meet Definition

Temple	Chester, PA
Case Western Reserve	Detroit
LSU – New Orleans	Baton Rouge
University of Vermont	Portland, ME

Not clear which campus is "main" and which is regional at time of study

University of Nevada	Reno or Las Vegas

Considered the "main" campus

Michigan State	Lansing

References

Association of American Medical Colleges. Minutes of the Proceedings, Sixty-Eighth Annual Meeting, October 21-23, 1957. *Journal of Medical Education.* 1958; 33: 59

Aronson LD, Murray RH. Internal medicine clerkship experience in community hospitals. In: Hunt AD, Weeks LE, eds. *Medical Education Since 1960: Marching to a Different Drummer.* East Lansing, Mich.: Michigan State University Foundation, 1979: 235-258.

Beljan JR. Living with community hospitals: Strategies to make the marriage work. In: Hunt AD, Weeks LE, eds. *Medical Education Since 1960: Marching to a Different Drummer.* East Lansing, Mich.: Michigan State University Foundation, 1979: 16-40.

Berg F. *The Role and Value of the University of Alabama School of Medicine Huntsville Regional Medical Campus and Tuscaloosa Regional Medical Campus.* Unpublished report, 2002.

Bolman LG, Deal TE. *Reframing Organizations: Artistry, Choice, and Leadership.* San Francisco: Jossey-Bass Publishers, 1991.

Bowers JZ, Purcell EF. *New Medical Schools at Home and Abroad: A Report of a Macy Conference.* New York: Josiah Macy Jr. Foundation, 1978.

Carnegie Commission on Higher Education. *Higher Education and the Nation's Health: Policies for Medical and Dental Education.* New York: McGraw-Hill Book Company, 1970.

Clark BR. *The Academic Life: Small Worlds, Different Worlds.* Princeton, N.J.: Carnegie Foundation for the Advancement of Teaching, 1987.

Costsonas NJ, Getz HG, Newman JI. The power inherent in equity. In: Hunt AD, Weeks LE, eds. *Medical Education Since 1960: Marching to a Different Drummer.* East Lansing, Mich.: Michigan State University Foundation, 1979: 41-56.

Creswell JW. A typology of multicampus systems. *Journal of Higher Education.* Jan-Feb 1985; 27: 26-37.

Deil R, Barshis D. Forging an institutional identity in a multicampus system. *Metropolitan Universities.* Fall 1996; 27: 27-40.

Dengerink HA. Institutional identify and organizational structure in multi-campus universities. *Metropolitan Universities.* Spring 2001; 12: 20-29.

Derzon RA. The marriage of medical schools and teaching hospitals. *Journal of Medical Education.* 1978; 53: 19-25.

Fields SA, Usatine R, Stearns JA, Toffler WL, Vinson DC. The use and compensation of community preceptors in U.S. medical schools. *Academic Medicine.* 1998; 73: 95-97.

Geiger RL. *Research and Relevant Knowledge: American Research Universities Since World War II.* New York: Oxford University Press, 1983.

Guba EG. *Toward a Methodology of Naturalistic Inquiry in Educational Evaluation.* Los Angeles: Center for the Study of Evaluation, UCLA Graduate School of Education, 1978.

Hunt AD. A time of change and reform in education. In: Hunt AD, Weeks LE, eds. *Medical Education Since 1960: Marching to a Different Drummer.* East Lansing, Mich.: Michigan State University Foundation, 1979: 2-10.

Jones RF, Sanderson SC. Clinical revenues used to support the academic mission of medical schools, 1992-3. *Academic Medicine.* 1996; 71: 299-307.

Keyes JA, Cohen PD, DeMuth GR, Rice WR. *Medical School-Clinical Affiliation Study Final Report.* Washington, D.C.: Division of Institutional Studies, Association of American Medical Colleges, 1977.

Lee EC, Bowen FM. *The Multicampus University: A Study of Academic Governance.* New York: McGraw-Hill Book Company, 1971.

Lewis IJ, Sheps CG. *The Sick Citadel: The American Academic Medical Center and the Public Interest.* Cambridge, Mass.: Oelgeschlager, Gunn, and Hain Publishers, 1983.

Lippard VW, Purcell EF, eds. *Case Histories of Ten New Medical Schools.* New York: Josiah Macy Jr. Foundation, 1972.

Ludmerer KM. *Time to Heal: American Medical Education from the Turn of the Century to the Era of Managed Care.* New York: Oxford University Press, 1999.

Merriam SB. *Qualitative Research and Case Study Applications in Education.* San Francisco: Jossey-Bass Publishers, 1998.

Miles MB, Huberman AM. *Qualitative Data Analysis.* 2nd ed. Thousand Oaks, Calif.: Sage Publications, 1994.

Nickerson M, Schaefer S. Autonomy and anonymity: Characteristics of branch campus faculty. *Metropolitan Universities.* Spring 2001; 12: 49-59.

Nutter D, Whitcomb M. *The AAMC Project on the Clinical Education of Medical Studies.* Washington, D.C.: Association of American Medical Colleges, 2001.

Parkin DL. The satellite campus: A collaborative model. *Planning for Higher Education.* Summer 1999; 27: 9-17.

Riesman D. *On Higher Education: The Academic Enterprise in an Era of Rising Student Consumerism.* San Francisco: Jossey-Bass Publishers, 1980.

Robinson L, ed. *AAMC Data Book: Statistical Information Related to Medical Schools and Teaching Hospitals.* Washington, D.C.: Association of American Medical Colleges, 2002.

Schofield JR. *New and Expanded Medical Schools, Mid-Century to the 1980s.* San Francisco: Jossey-Bass, 1984.

Shannon JA. The advancement of medical research: A twenty-year view of the role of the National Institutes of Health. *Journal of Medical Education.* 1967; 42: 97-108.

Smith R. Governance and corporate identity in network universities. *Journal of Tertiary Educational Administration.* May 1992; 14: 5-10.

SUNY Upstate Medical Center, Binghamton Clinical Campus. *Narrative Database for LCME Limited Site Visit.* September 17-19, 1990.

Swick HM. *Medical Education at Regional Campuses: A Status Report.* Unpublished report. January 2000.

Surgeon General's Consultant Group on Medical Education. *Physicians for a Growing America.* Washington, D.C.: Public Health Service, U.S. Department of Health, Education, and Welfare, 1959. Public Health Service Publication No. 709.

Watt JM, Dubach S, Madison K, Peck M. *A Study of Medical Schools Operating Geographically Separated Campuses.* Corte Madera, Calif.: Lewin-VHI, Inc., December 1993.

Watts EM. Governance beyond the individual campus. *Academe.* Sept-Oct 1991; 77: 28-30, 32-33.

Yin RK. *Case Study Research: Design and Methods.* 2nd ed. Thousand Oaks, Calif.: Sage Publication, 1994.

Index

AAMC Project on the Clinical Education of Medical Students (2001), 2, 37, 39, 40
academic departments, 58-60
academic medical centers, culture of, 41-42, 52
area health education centers (AHECs), 8

Bane Report, 5-6
basic science campuses, 3, 65
biomedical research, 11-12, 26-27
branch campus
    See clinical campus
    See also basic science campuses

Carnegie Commission on Higher Education, 6, 7-8, 11
clinical campus
    administrative structure of, 24-27
    benefits of, 33-36, 37-42, 63
    community and, 35
    deans of, 26-27
    definition of, 2-4
    drawbacks of, 42-44
    faculty at, 30-32, 46-49
    for expanding medical school enrollment, 2
    history of, 5-13
    hospitals and, 34-35
    organization of, 15, 51-62
    medical education at, 28-29, 37-46
    primary care emphasis of, 7, 8
    reasons for, 33-36
    research at, 27
    student recruitment to, 44-46
    year of founding, 23
clerkship directors, 39, 60-61
community-based medical schools, 6-7, 13, 14
culture, research, 11-12, 42-43
curriculum management, 60-61

departments
    See academic departments
definition of regional campus, 2-4
distance, impediments of, 55-57
distributed model of education, 1, 11

education
    See medical education

faculty, 30-32, 46-49
faculty development, 48-49

geographically separated campus
    See clinical campus
graduate medical education, 7, 10, 28

Health Professions Assistance Act, 5-7
healthcare
    changing delivery of, 9
    right to, 7-8
historical context of regional campuses, 5-13

innovations in medical education, 37-39
institutional relationships, 51-62

Jefferson, Thomas, 63-64

Liaison Committee on Medical Education, 3, 60-61

"major" hospital affiliate, 3
medical education, 28-29, 37-46
    innovations in, 37-39
    technology and, 44

medical school, 1-2
    class size, 6, 9
    relationships with hospitals, 4, 9, 14-15, 25-26, 34-35, 51
medical students
    education experiences of, 2, 28-29, 37-46, 63
    recruitment of, 44-45
Medicare, 7-8

National Institutes of Health, 11-12, 27

patient volume, 9, 33-34, 40
physician supply, 2, 5-7, 33
Physicians for a Growing America, 5-6
primary care emphasis, 7-8, 33

recruitment of medical students, 44-45
regional campus
    See clinical campus
regional deans, 2, 26-27, 51-54
research "culture", 42-43
residency programs, 7, 10, 28, 43

satellite campus
    See clinical campus
symbolism, 54-56

technology, influence on medical education, 44
tenure, at regional campuses 47-48